Hello and welcome! I'm thrilled you've joined us.

Dive into a world of health, happiness and joy with *"Splash*Dance: What a Feeling!"* Discover how aqua fitness and positive psychology can empower you to flourish and feel fantastic. For a deeper splash into our aquatic adventures, including visual illustrations of *Splash*Dance choreography, moving musical playlists, and science-backed tips to lift your mood, give you positive energy and boost your confidence, visit my website, **ElaineOBrienPhD.com**.

Let me know how I can help you look and feel great.

You can reach me at **Dr.ElaineOB@gmail.com**—just put *"Splash-Dance"* in your subject line. Here's to riding the waves of well-being and happiness together.

With heartfelt appreciation,

Dr. Elaine O'Brien

SPLASH DANCE

WHAT A FEELING!

Aqua Fitness Meets Positive Psychology

DR. ELAINE O'BRIEN

LiveLifeHappy Publishing

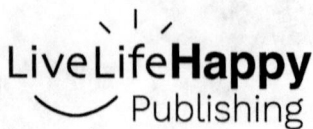

Library of Congress Cataloging-in-Publication Data

Dr. Elaine O'Brien

SplashDance: What a Feeling!

Categories: Health, Fitness & Dieting > Exercise & Fitness > Physical Therapy > Aquatic Exercise > Self-Help > Stress Management > Personal Transformation > Happiness > Sports & Outdoors > Water Sports > Swimming > Psychology & Counseling > Applied Psychology > Positive Psychology > Medical eBooks > Special Topics (Geriatrics) > Sports Medicine

ISBN E-Book: 978-1-990461-82-8

ISBN Paperback: 978-1-990461-81-1

Cover, Photography, and Creative Design: Lianna Tarantin

Copy Editor: Sean O'Brien

Live Life Happy Publishing

PUBLISHER'S NOTE & AUTHOR DISCLAIMER

"...I think of you every day. Now that I have converted all my daily exercises into the pool: 20 minutes of jogging and stretching, I welcome your suggestions further."

— Sent via email from the legendary, Dr. Martin Seligman, founder of Positive Psychology, mentor, and cherished friend, who inspired me to bring this book to fruition. My hope is that it can help lead you to flourishing health and happiness.

Dedication

To my Mother, Frances Perrotta, and Nunni, Anna Richichi, for ensuring I learned to swim.

To my sweetheart of a Dad, Armando Perrotta, who played in the pool and swam with my little brother Mike and me, and who inspired me to love the water.

To Lianna Tarantin, my brilliant, beautiful darling daughter, creative director, water ballerina, Pisces aqua baby, and SplashDance photographer.

To Sean O'Brien, my darling mate, and copy editor, so happy I met you, Neighbor, five blocks from the shore in historic Ocean Grove. Here's to you, Love, and 25 more!

CONTENTS

INTRODUCTION

Hello and welcome! I'm Dr. Elaine O'Brien, and it's my honor to introduce you to "*Splash*Dance: What a Feeling!" With a PhD in Kinesiology, focusing on the Psychology of Human Movement earned in 2015, I have had the joy of teaching rhythmic dance and exercise both on land and in the water for over two decades. For me, aqua fitness is more than just a profession—it's a personal voyage through health, healing, discovery, and joy. It has also been a powerful way to forge positive, vibrant connections.

Teaching in the water has been some of the most rewarding, exhilarating and fun-filled experiences of my career. I am thrilled to share this book with you, and to invite you to revel in the enlivening and joy-filled world of *Splash*Dance. Whether you're looking to enhance your physical health, find emotional balance, or connect with others, *Splash*Dance offers you a welcoming space to thrive. My aim and mission is to help you protect and improve your muscular endurance, strength, aerobic capacity, flexibility, agility, balance, coordination, and power, while having the most fun possible.

So, What is *Splash*Dance?

*Splash*Dance combines the transformative properties of aqua fitness with the uplifting principles of positive psychology. My groundbreaking program transcends traditional aqua fitness by integrating rhythmic Vertical Aqua Fitness (VAF) with scientifically backed techniques to enhance your health and vitality. This innovative training method is performed upright in the buoyant, soothing embrace of water. *Splash*Dance offers a personal and invigorating experience, dedicated to enhancing well-being through rhythmic movement to music, applying positive leadership, and connecting individuals within a welcoming atmosphere.

Immerse yourself in this fun, effective, and inspiring training that not only elevates your physical health but also enhances your mood, leaving you invigorated long after you've left the pool. This unique blend of exciting aqua dynamics, positive psychology, and positive movement science creates a transformative approach to health, healing, and flourishing well-being, while countering symptoms of inactivity, depression, and loneliness.

*Splash*Dance also serves as an excellent, dynamic form of cross-conditioning for athletes and enthusiasts across all sports. The water's supportive nature allows you to safely experiment with balance and agility exercises without the risk of falling, enabling powerful movements against the resistance of a fluid environment.

Unlike traditional swimming, which is predominantly horizontal, *Splash*Dance's routines are mostly performed vertically, meaning you don't need to get your hair or face wet while engaging in this enlivening fitness discipline. This book will guide you through the why and how of using *Splash*Dance to achieve a healthier, happier, confident, and more joyful state of being.

Celebrating Mind & Body Wisdom For Preventative Health and Holistic Well-Being

How would you like to add more vitality to your life? Would you enjoy a fitness adventure that is not only effective but also joyful and rejuvenating? *Splash*Dance is your ideal sustainable fitness prescription.

This program celebrates preventative health and holistic well-being with every purposeful, determined movement. Performed in water of varying depths, and for the dancer, non-dancer, swimmer, and non-swimmer alike, *Splash*Dance will help you look and feel great.

A Social Prescription for Fitness and Flourishing

Drawing on decades of experience teaching, training instructors, researching, presenting, and actively participating, I've both immersed myself and witnessed the transformative power of aqua exercise. The scientifically backed, multi-dimensional benefits of *Splash*Dance offer a superior social fitness prescription, delivering psychological, cognitive, physical rewards.

*Splash*Dance allies with Dr. Martin Seligman's PERMA model of well-being—Positivity, Engagement, Relationships, Meaning, and Achievement—and is enhanced further by other positive psychological elements including flow, self-determination (autonomy, competence, relatedness), gratitude, character strengths, and communitas, fostering a sense of community well-being.

FUNctional Fitness and Aging Healthy and Well

Whether you're a seasoned athlete or just beginning your fitness journey, *Splash*Dance provides adaptable, powerful, yet gentle, aerobic cross-training. Delight in the dynamic moves, engaging choreography, and a buoyant atmosphere. Each session enhances your energy, strength, flexibility, agility, and balance—key components for aging healthy and well. This form of FUNctional Fitness, powered by the joy of movement, offers purposeful and pleasurable activity in a fluid environment.

A Groundbreaking Exploration

"*Splash*Dance: What a Feeling!" is a groundbreaking exploration into the world of aquatic fitness, offering a fresh perspective on exercise that combines the joy of movement with the therapeutic qualities of water. The book is thoughtfully divided into three different aspects of the *Splash*Dance experience and its broader implications.

Part One of the book lays the foundation of the *Splash*Dance program, offering you a detailed guide to the mechanics, benefits, and joys of this innovative, mostly vertical aqua exercise regimen. From easy-to-follow, challenging choreography to the underlying physics that enhance training's effectiveness, this section is enriched with fun facts and insightful tips. It serves as both a how-to manual for enthusiasts and a compelling argument for why aqua fitness is a transformative experience that leverages the natural resistance and buoyancy of water to foster physical and mental well-being.

Part Two shifts the focus towards the potential of aqua fitness as a promising career and calling. It delves into the leadership aspects required to lead the *Splash*Dance method, providing valuable tips on class formatting, effective cueing, and leadership. This section is an indispensable resource for the enthusiasts as well as current and aspiring fitness professionals who see themselves as future leaders in the aqua fitness industry, equipping them with the necessary skills and insights to excel and inspire.

Part Three offers an optimistic gaze towards the future, emphasizing the role of *Splash*Dance in addressing and mitigating contemporary challenges such as physical inactivity and social isolation, along with fostering a narrative around aging healthfully and well. It expands to discuss the profound impact of integrating positive psychology through strength-based approaches and the potential of *Splash*Dance to serve as a social prescription for a healthier, more connected society, as well as individual growth.

By weaving together practical instruction, leadership training, and visionary outlooks, "*Splash*Dance: What a Feeling!" invites you to dive deeply into the transformative power of aquatic fitness, making it an essential read for anyone passionate about fostering health and happiness through innovative, positive aqua movement.

Find Your Purpose and Radiant Well-Being

Explore vertical aqua fitness as you dive deep into the art, science, and biomechanics of this delightful discipline. Draw inspiration from practical tips, groundbreaking research, and personal stories of hopeful change. This innovative, enjoyable, and focused training synchronizes with the rhythm of positivity, offering well-being that radiates vitality and joy. Together, let's navigate the currents of life, finding strength, harmony, and purpose in every motion.

Let's get on deck—it's time to *Splash*Dance!

PART ONE

Aqua Fitness Meets Positive Psychology

CHAPTER 1

Splash into Vitality - Vertical Aqua Fitness and Positive Transformation

"Dance with the waves,
Move with the sea,
Let the rhythms of the water,
Set your soul free."

– Christy Ann Martine, Canadian Poet,
Mom, Nature Lover.

Delight into a world where water isn't just a place to swim—it's a vibrant, dynamic medium for transformation and vitality. Welcome to "*Splash*Dance: What a Feeling!" Immerse yourself in the exhilarating world of Vertical Aqua Fitness (VAF), where the uplifting buoyancy of water synergizes with the vibrant energy of a variety of fortifying movements in the pool. This groundbreaking program combines aqua dynamics with positive psychology, offering an innovative approach to enhancing health, boosting fitness, and invigorating vitality. Engage your core, improve your balance, and embrace a workout that's as gentle or intense as you need it to be.

Are you ready for more energy and joy in your life? Are you looking to infuse more zest into your life? Would you like to boost your strength, flexibility, or simply lighten your mood? Whether you're aiming to enhance your health, manage your weight, or cross-train for athletic pursuits, or if you're seeking to elevate your vitality, strengthen your body, or brighten your mood, SplashDance offers a fun, supportive, and effective workout regimen for preventative health and holistic well-being. It's perfect for:

- **Dancers and non-dancers alike**
- **Swimmers and non-swimmers**
- **Individuals of any fitness level**

*Splash*Dance invites you to revel in:

- **Improved flexibility**
- **Enhanced strength**
- **Greater endurance**
- **Better balance**
- **Robust cardiovascular health — all within the supportive embrace of water.**

My program, the *Splash*Dance method, is an inclusive program in that it welcomes participants of all ages to explore a variety of movements. From gentle stretches and spirited jumps to intricate moves, we offer you easy-to-follow formations and great music across diverse genres, *Splash*Dance is an exceptional form of dynamic cross-training suitable for novices, athletes, and fitness enthusiasts alike. The water's supportive nature allows for safe, bold experimentation with balance and agility exercises, enabling powerful movements against the unique resistance of a fluid environment.

Leveraging the Water's Magical Properties

Unlike traditional swimming, which primarily involves horizontal movements, aqua fitness embraces the vertical dimension to harness the physics of aqua dynamics. This unique positioning allows you to maximize the complexity and benefits of your workouts in a setting that integrates both non-impact (deep-water fitness training) and low-impact exercises (training about chest height depth), where one foot may remain on the ground. This vertical approach is effective, gentle, and powerfully innovative.

The comprehensive methods include rhythmic aerobics, strength and resistance training, flexibility, variable and high-intensity interval training (HIIT), relaxations and movements borrowed from Pilates, yoga, martial arts, sports, and dance. The empowering cross-training enhances your muscular strength, fuels your energy, and endurance, all while being gentle on your joints.

Aligning with the principles of positive psychology, which is broadly, the science of happiness, well-being, and flourishing, *Splash*Dance offers a holistic approach: mind-body wisdom. This book will expertly guide you through the 'why' and the 'how' of utilizing the dynamic and beneficial forces of water for your whole well-being.

Embark on this aquatic adventure and take a fulfilling step forward toward flourishing in every aspect of your life—physical, neurological, psychological, emotional, and social. *Splash*Dance is more than just exercise; it's a playful, impactful path to positive health and thriving. Get ready to embrace a healthier, more vibrant, and joyous state of being as you discover the possibilities and power of *Splash*Dance.

Cheers to a healthier, happier you!

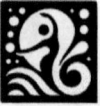

Questions for Reflection and Positive Action

Vitality through *Splash*Dance: How might *Splash*Dance bring more vitality into your life?

Supportive Water Environment: How might a supportive and risk-free water environment change your approach to physical fitness?

Exploration and Achievement: What would you be excited to explore or achieve on your *Splash*Dance journey?

CHAPTER 2

The Ripple Effect - Tides of Growth and Positive Personal Changes

In this chapter, we explore the transformative power of aqua fitness. This begins with a thoughtful note from Dr. Martin Seligman, the father of positive psychology, about his new exploration of aqua fitness and its power and healing embrace. Further, we delve into serendipity and inspiring stories on overcoming physical and emotional challenges. These triumphant narratives celebrate not just survival but thriving, marked by strength, joy, and community.

"I Welcome Your Suggestions."

Cherished mentor and friend, Dr. Martin Seligman, affectionately known as the "father of positive psychology," has expressed a new-found interest in the benefits of aqua fitness, writing to me recently, "...I think of you every day. Now that I have converted all my daily exercises into the pool: 20 minutes of jogging and stretching, I welcome your suggestions further."

Marty, thank you for your brilliance, for the hopeful and agentic science of positive psychology, and for inspiring the "suggestions" in this book: to have fun, and to move well, and more in the pool. I recently saw Marty in his exquisite "Marty Seligman" rose garden, adjacent to his pool; he is strong, looking fitter, and seems quite happy about adding aqua exercise into his life!

This timely validation means the world because I believe *SplashDance has* the ability to lead people toward flourishing, health, and happiness. It's a thrill to share the science, applications, and my experiences around the pool with you.

Serendipity: My Personal Journey Teaching "Land" and Then Aqua Fitness

I started to teach aerobic dance (on land) at the beginning of the fitness revolution, auditioning as an "Aerobics Instructor" with Roger's Dance Studio, Westfield, NJ. Rogers, Dennis, and Jackie, were brilliant teachers, who were affiliated with the prestigious Imperial Society for Ballroom Dance. I was a non-dancer, with no experience, and frankly the worst trainee in my *Aerobics 'n Rhythm* training class; Jackie and Dennis told me they "gave me a shot because I had a nice personality." I was out of shape and uncoordinated. But I loved it, and I loved the music, the energy, the aerobic dance, the teaching, and the potential positive outcomes, so I persevered. It did change my life, and just saying, if I can do it, anyone can.

My personal journey into teaching aqua exercises began unexpectedly—serendipitously, you might say. I was a student in a Water Aerobics class when, after three sessions, our instructor suddenly quit. I found myself thrust into co-teaching along with my pool classmate, friend, and fellow *Aerobics 'n Rhythm* dance/exercise leader at Shore Fitness, Carol Dunphy. Encouraged by our aqua group, Carol and I took the plunge, teaching the classes at Avon Pool that summer. Those early days were filled with practice, play, and plenty of laughter, igniting a deep-seated passion within me.

Determined to keep learning, I sought out training, tools, and a certification from the Aquatics Exercise Association, founded and led by industry leader, Ruth Sova. I studied the research, and then confidently designed, taught, and presented pool fitness programs utilizing the best practices of Aqua Physics, that I examined with a fellow fitness professional who was an athlete and a mechanical engineer.

My goal was to create innovative and effective methods for fun, individual, and group water exercises. I developed *Splash*Dance, a rhythmic movement program that boosts well-being and strengthens community ties. This program promotes physical activity and positive connections, enriching vitality, and enjoyment for participants.

Teaching *Splash*Dance is my harmonious passion. Seeing the positive effects my aqua fitness training has on people, both individually and in a group, is heartening.

Embracing Aqua Dynamics, Psychology, and Leadership in a Fluid Environment

As I moved from novice to expert, my professional path took a significant turn. I continued my love of teaching along with the excitement of training fellow instructors. A high point was presenting for the first Aquatics Exercise Association conference, and then for the IDEA Health and Fitness Association World Congress. At IDEA, I led a session on Aqua Dynamics, including my research and applications of aqua fitness leadership, psychology, and physics in a fluid environment, which was a new concept in the field. It was a thrill to be at the forefront of aqua fitness innovation, leadership and training. The best part was to be able to inspire and train leaders who would take the knowledge and lead many more people to greater health, fitness and community well-being.

A Phenomenon of Self-Determination and Transformative Positive Health

Among the most rewarding aspects of my career has been witnessing my students' profound transformations. Here are two stories that are poignant testaments to the healing and growth that aqua fitness and positive psychology can facilitate.

Overcoming Trauma: Building Neural Connections and Pathways To Healing

On a sunny summer day, a woman, Ms. S, approached the pool deck with cautious steps. A brain injury had disrupted her neural pathways, impacting her speech, gait, and mobility. Her legs, also affected, offered little support. She told me the story about her injuries and trauma, and how she had a very difficult time exercising on land. In the pool, we trained and played together, with a gentle yet strengthening approach to help and heal her. Eventually, we added more complexity: strength training, aerobics as water walking, in shallow (chest height) and deep water. Over months of perseverance and dedication, she began to reconnect with her brain and her body in extraordinary ways. The water served as a vital link in lowering her trauma, both physically and emotionally.

Over time, she was able to make valuable connections to her health and healing via the therapeutic aqua fitness training and her own inspiring positive self-determination. She also lost 100 pounds. Members of our program admired and cheered on her courage and dedication.

She ultimately gained confidence, fitness, and is a lifelong friend. Through attending a simple aqua fitness program, my cherished student was able to transform her life and inspire others. Despite facing further personal tragedies and losses, she remains a beacon of hope, love, and gratitude, her story is a powerful reminder of the indomitable strength and resilience inherent in all of us.

My student friend has repeatedly said I "saved her life." Reflecting on this, I realize the immense power of creating a welcoming, loving, kind environment to facilitate healing. My aim to set a warm and encouraging tone played a role in her journey. Truly, she is my inspiration. A living example of Positive Self-Determination Theory, which values growth through autonomy, relationships, and mastery, she made the courageous decision to step into the pool, build nurturing friendships, and achieve a new level of independence and vitality.

This story honors the human spirit, celebrating her and her journey, and the transformative healing benefits of aqua fitness and its potential for renewal. There is joy that lies within our embrace of water.

Trish Sullivan: Finding Empowerment and Renewal in the Waters of Aqua Fitness

My fellow aqua fitness classmate, Trish Sullivan, has another remarkable story about building neural connections. Hers is also a remarkable transformation I've witnessed firsthand; it is a journey of recovery and empowerment. Trish has also experienced deep "meaning-making."

This refers to how we as people interpret and give significance to our life experiences, shaping our beliefs, values, and understanding of the world.

A finance professional and mother of two, Trish enjoyed a vibrant life filled with family, work, and leisure—until one ordinary day turned catastrophic.

While walking her dog with her husband, a freak accident occurred—a dead Sycamore tree suddenly fell, striking Trish on the head. This severe injury led to cognitive losses, balance issues, anxiety, tinnitus, and significant disruptions to her finances and identity. Yet, it is in the buoyant sanctuary of the pool at the Neptune Aquatics Center that Trish is finding her path to healing.

When Trish agreed to my interview, I had no idea of her suffering. I wanted to talk with Trish because she seemed to be enjoying the classes and music so much. Her dedication and cheerful demeanor intrigued me. When we met, she shared her harrowing yet inspiring story. Despite the severe trauma she endured, Trish spoke of aqua fitness with passion, declaring, "It transformed my life for the better."

Encouraged by her neurologist to try aqua fitness as part of her rehabilitation, Trish discovered more than just physical therapy in the water; she found her "Happy Place." Only six months into her aqua fitness journey, she has experienced remarkable improvements—increased confidence, better sleep, and enhanced overall well-being. Trish is finding happiness, along with greater strength, tone, and energy as she powerfully and joyfully moves through the water each class.

Trish's story is another testament to the restorative power of aqua fitness, not only as a physical regimen but also as an empowering emotional and psychological uplift. We also see her neural connections being reestablished through the aqua movement, music, and social dimension.

"Aqua fitness is a win-win, a lifesaver," she says, grateful for the empowerment she feels every time she enters the water. Just like my previous student, Trish's recovery highlights how aqua fitness can offer a new lease on life for those recovering from injuries, proving once again that we must always remember the profound impact of kindness and support in our shared journeys of living and healing. Trish, thanks for your smile.

If these two inspiring women with severe brain injury are experiencing far-reaching, positively remarkable healing benefits via aqua fitness, can you imagine how it benefits someone neurologically, cognitively, and psychologically without a trauma?

Resilience Ripples: Sharlene Langner's Triumph Over Depression and Cancer

I met Sharlene Langner when we were helping a fellow student retrieve her aqua glove in the deep end of the pool. We started chatting, and Sharlene shared her poignant, inspiring, and powerful story with me. Three years ago, Sharlene also discovered the therapeutic embrace of the water at Neptune Aquatics Center.

Suffering from major depressive disorder and suicide ideation, Sharlene found the pool to be a place that was soothing, and that provided her with physical and social connections. A non-swimmer, she started aqua fitness classes, and at age 65, she learned to swim. Sharlene overcame her fears, and over time, one lap became one mile! She also learned to dive.

Sharlene spoke about the benefits of the water, saying it's the best exercise, I enjoy it, and I'm committed to it, saying, "It changed my life." For Sharlene, the pool became more than a place to exercise; it became a sanctuary offering physical, emotional, and social nourishment. She said, "The water is healing. There's no competition, and no one can see you from the neck down."

Her journey took an unexpected turn when she was diagnosed with cancer. Sharlene asked her doctors about returning to the pool almost immediately after her diagnosis, eager to reclaim the strength and peace she found in the water. Aqua Fitness did more than just strengthen her body; it bolstered her spirit and confidence, empowering her to make significant life changes, including leaving a high-pressure career as a corporate leadership development professional to pursue a life that truly resonated with her soul.

Sharlene credits her remarkable recovery from both depression and cancer to "her psychologist, psychiatrist, and the pool." Her resilience, attitude, and transformative experiences in the water are a testament to her courage and strength.

As she navigates the challenges of life, Sharlene remains anchored by her belief in the healing power of water, sharing, "I love water exercise; the benefits last all day." And "I never worry in the water."

Sharlene's story is a beacon of hope and resilience. It's about embracing change with grace and finding strength in vulnerability. She sincerely wishes her narrative will inspire others and offer a message of positive self-determination. Sharlene's story is not just about overcoming, but thriving—not just surviving, but flourishing with kindness and an unyielding spirit of bravery, perseverance, and possibility. Thank you, Sharlene.

Resilient Well-Being

Aqua Fitness has helped me. After being gutted by a year marked with heart-wrenching sadness and tragedy, I committed to partici-pating in a variety of fitness classes 3-5 times/week at the Neptune Aquatics Center pool in Neptune, New Jersey. I am happy being a student again. What a game-changer. Even though I love it, I don't always want to go to class, (and can come up with lots of excuses NOT to go). I persevere and I <u>always</u> feel better as soon as I hit the water, AND afterward. In comparing notes with fellow students, Trish and Sharlene included, there's a sense we are experiencing an upward spiral of positive emotional health by virtue of our aqua fitness training, and the many physical benefits.

Looking Ahead with Excitement

As I now prepare to teach my *Splash*Dance method at Fairway Mews' Community Pool for the 20th year, I'm reflecting on how an aqua fitness program can transform lives. *Splash*Dance is more than an exercise; it's a rhythmic celebration of movement and community. It enhances muscular strength, aerobic capacity, and flexibility, and equally importantly, it fosters emotional and social well-being.

I spoke with Paula Toledo, a "Social Prescriptions" expert, a brilliant musician, and my fellow MAPP friend. Based on our conversation, it is clear *Splash*Dance boosts positive social connections, while also reducing the risk of diseases of loneliness and inactivity; *Splash*Dance is a Social Prescription that matters.

This narrative of healing change, inspiration, community, and joy in aqua fitness is an invitation for you to discover your own path in the comforting, yet powerful embrace of water. Join me in this rhythmic exploration of aqua fitness, where each splash can bring us closer to positive health and happiness.

A Call and Calling to *Splash*Dance

Thank you for joining me on this personal and professional journey through aqua fitness, *Splash*Dance, a sensory celebration. It is a movement that offers a space where physical health, emotional balance, and community connections can thrive. Let's dive in.

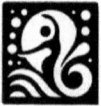

Questions for Reflection and Positive Action

Reflect on Your Journey: What goals or challenges might encourage you to try new forms of exercise like *Splash*Dance?

Explore the Power of Community: Knowing that being part of a positive community can lead you to greater well-being, what steps can you take to enhance your social connectivity?

Commit to Trying New Things: Inspired by Dr. Martin Seligman's embrace of aquatic exercises, how might you apply aqua fitness to enhance not just your physical health but also your emotional and mental well-being?

CHAPTER 3

Aqua Powered Fitness Meets Positive Psychology: Currents of Joy

"If there is magic on this planet,
it is contained in water."

- Loren Eiseley, Anthropologist, Science Writer, Educator

At its heart, SplashDance is not just an aquatic exercise; it's a celebration of well-being, using the rhythmic power of water to propel individuals and communities toward greater health and happiness. Aligned with Dr. Martin Seligman's PERMA model, this program encapsulates the essence of flourishing by fostering positive emotions, engagement, relationships, meaning, and achievement. Join us as we explore how each *Splash*Dance session not only enhances physical fitness but also enriches lives and holistic well-being.

PERMA Well-Being: Seligman's Model of Flourishing

At its core, *Splash*Dance is an individual and community-based method of valuing people's well-being, movement, and positive connections in the context of a fluid environment with the ultimate goal of "moving people toward positive health and happiness." *Splash*Dance energizes with a rhythmic synergy of music and motion, fostering an environment ripe for personal and community growth and joy.

The *Splash*Dance program design embraces with Seligman's *PERMA* model of flourishing.

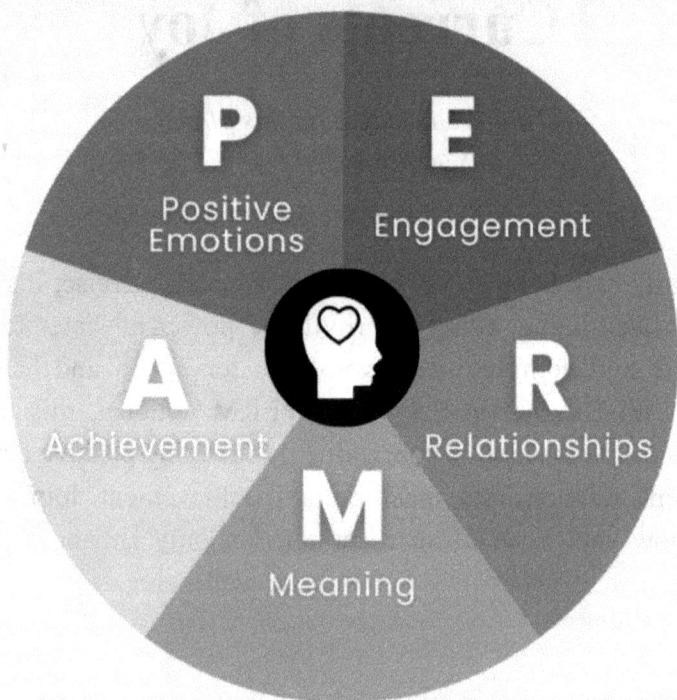

Each *Splash*Dance session encourages **positive emotions**, enhances **engagement**, primes **relationships**, offers a chance for **meaning,** and has you leaving your training feeling proud of your **achievements.** Seligman's (2011) "PERMA" is a theoretical model of happiness, well-being, and flourishing:

1. **Positive Emotions**: *Splash*Dance fosters an environment filled with lightness and laughter, essential for cultivating positive emotions, such as hope, happiness and joy. These positive emotions broaden your attention, cognition and action. This creates possibilities for building your personal, intellectual, social and psychological resources. The buoyant nature of water exercise naturally elevates mood and reduces stress, helping you to feel more optimistic and energized during and after each session.

2. **Engagement**: The immersive nature of rhythmic aquatic movements allows you to lose yourself, fully absorbing yourself in the joy of the moment and the physicality of your movements. In a *Splash*Dance experience, there's also an opportunity to prime deep engagement, often referred to as "flow."

3. **Relationships**: As a communal activity, *Splash*Dance supports and strengthens social connections. The shared experience of moving together in water creates a sense of camaraderie and community, fostering supportive and positive relationships, which can elevate social well-being.

4. **Meaning**: Being part of *Splash*Dance offers more than just physical benefits; it provides you with a sense of purpose and belonging. Enhancing your personal and communal well-being lends a meaningful aspect, as you feel you are part of something larger than yourself.

5. **Achievement**: Every session of *Splash*Dance gives you the opportunity to set and reach goals, whether they are related to fitness, coordination, or personal growth. The sense of accomplishment

derived from mastering new moves, improving endurance, and contributing to a group effort fuels a sense of achievement.

*Splash*Dance is not just about physical health; it's a comprehensive model for flourishing that supports whole well-being and mind-body wisdom.

Harnessing Agency: How *Splash*Dance Empowers and Inspires

Aqua fitness revitalizes not only the body but also the mind, nurturing a belief in personal efficacy as you observe your own progress and abilities in the water. This dual empowerment—both physical and psychological—bolsters optimism, inspiring confidence that the benefits gained in the pool, like enhanced strength and endurance, will extend into other aspects of your life. *Splash*Dance inspires positive transformation and enhances your agency, empowering you with resources to help you fulfill your potential.

Furthermore, "*Splash*Dance" taps into the power of imagination, enabling you to envision and realize a healthier, more joyful existence. Psychologist, Martin Seligman highlights that when we recognize our agency, we are more inclined to adopt behaviors that foster well-being. Within the vibrancy of "*Splash*Dance", this translates into participation in an activity that not only supports but also uplifts and boosts your resilience and creativity. "SplashDance" is a celebration of human potential and a direct application of positive psychology's PERMA model of flourishing, cultivating Pleasant emotions, Engagement, supportive Relationships, Meaning, and Achievement—all within the invigorating and joyful realm of water.

Whole Well-being Through *Splash*Dance

Immerse yourself in the multifaceted benefits of *Splash*Dance, where each movement propels you toward enhanced physical, psychological, and cognitive well-being. Discover the holistic advantages of integrating this dynamic water workout into your lifestyle:

Physical Health: Delight in cardiovascular conditioning, muscle strengthening and toning, agility, and flexibility. *Splash*Dance harnesses the unique properties of water to deliver a comprehensive and enjoyable workout that effectively boosts overall fitness.

Psychological Benefits: *Splash*Dance doesn't just condition your body—it elevates your spirit. Enjoy mood enhancement, distress reduction, positive energy, and flourishing mental well-being.

Cognitive Gains: Engage with the benefits of increased oxygen flow to the brain and enhanced neuroplasticity (brain changing), and neurogenesis (brain building) benefits through *Splash*Dance's rhythmic cardiovascular movements. This joyful fluid activity nurtures your brain's health and executive functions.

Gratitude: Recognized as a transcendent strength, gratitude involves acknowledging the goodness in one's life. Positive movement, like in *Splash*Dance primes feelings of thankfulness and appreciation.

Self-Determination Theory: The *Splash*Dance program is meticulously designed to meet your psychological needs for autonomy, competence, and relatedness. Choose your movements within a supportive framework, master various aqua fitness techniques, and connect with a community that fosters a sense of belonging. This enriching environment boosts motivation and enriches your experience with *Splash*Dance.

Finding Flow with *Splash*Dance

Dive deep and lose yourself in the experience. The concept of "flow," as articulated by the late, great psychologist Dr. Mihaly Csikszentmihalyi, describes a state of profound immersion and engagement in an activity, marked by fulfilling enjoyment and a loss of time awareness. Explore how *Splash*Dance can facilitate these beneficial psychological flow states.

How *Splash*Dance Facilitates Flow

*Splash*Dance beautifully leverages the concept of psychological flow, creating a deeply engaging aquatic experience that enhances both mental and physical health. In flow, there is a perfect balance between challenge and skill, making each movement feel rewarding and enjoyable. This optimal engagement not only boosts psychological well-being by reducing stress and enhancing happiness but also encourages long-term commitment to the activity. By transforming exercise into a joyous celebration, *Splash*Dance promotes sustained health behaviors and habits, making it a powerful incentive and tool for holistic because you get to:

1. **Engage in Enjoyable Elements:** The unique environment provided by water adds a novel element and complexity. The sensation of moving through water is refreshing, playful, and stimulating, which can readily lead to a flow state.

2. **Create Adjustable Resistance:** Water provides natural, adjustable resistance based on the type of movement, speed, lever length, or use of equipment. Tailor challenges to match your skill level, and as you become more adept, increase the challenges to prime flow.

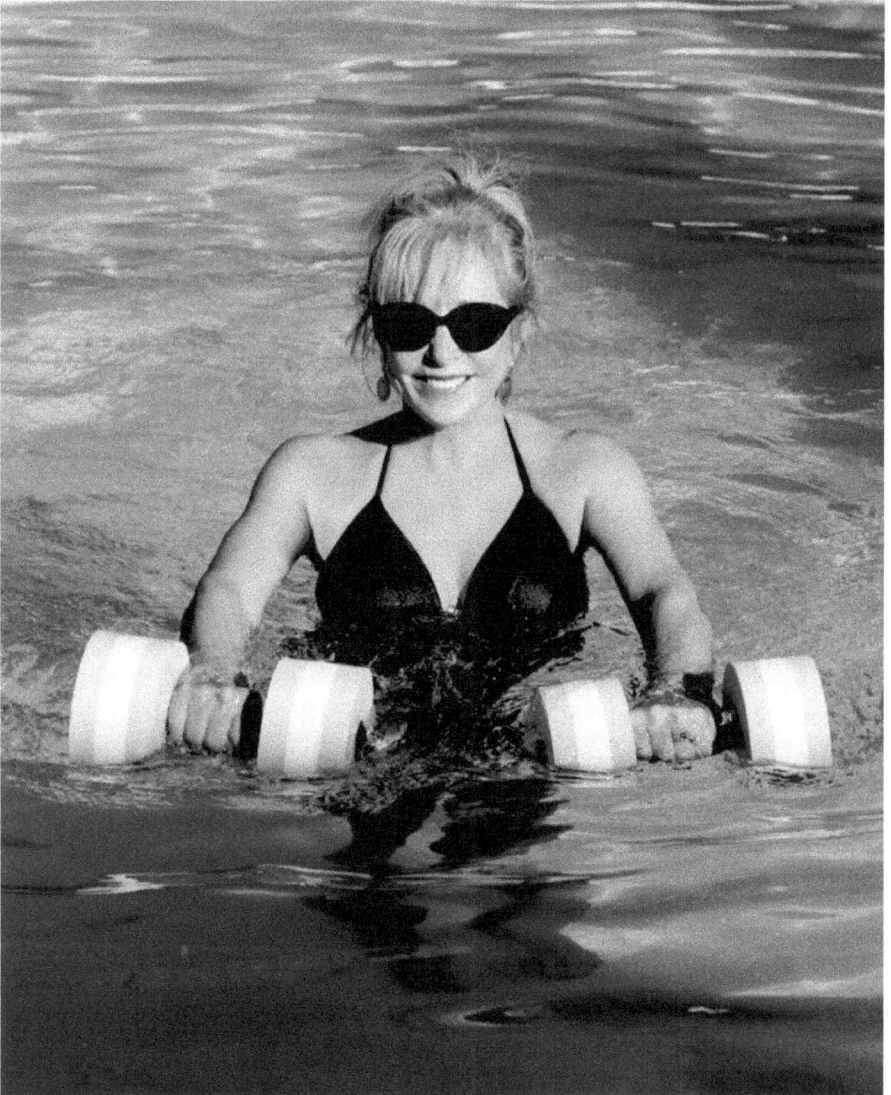

Photo: Lianna Tarantin

2. **Enhance Your Focus:** Aqua fitness training demands concentration to maintain balance and coordinate movements in a fluid medium. Water minimizes distractions, allowing for full immersion, both literally and figuratively.

3. **Savor the Immediate Physical Feedback:** As you perform different movements, the immediate feedback loop from the water helps you stay engaged. You feel the resistance, adjust your effort and technique accordingly, and maintain flow.

4. **Experience Confidence and Control:** The buoyancy of water may boost your confidence, encouraging you to experiment with the intensity, variations, control, and complexity of movements.

5. **Transcend a Time Transformation:** A hallmark of being in flow is altered time perception. When engaged in enjoyable yet challenging activities like *Splash*Dance, you might find that time seems to pass quickly, a common indicator of the flow state.

6. **Enhance Flow For Holistic Health and Fitness**: According to Csikszenmihalyi, adults who limit movement experiences reduce their potential for flow and run the risk of cardiovascular disease, lung disease, and Type 1 diabetes, as well as high blood pressure, stroke, disability and depression. Activating flow supports well-being.

*Splash*Dance isn't just a fitness program—it's a holistic approach to thriving. We are happy to invite you to explore your potential and enjoy a fuller, more vibrant life. *Splash*Dance is your chance to boost your mind, body, heart, brain, and soul all in the medium of refreshing, exhilarating, supportive, and comforting water.

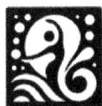

Questions for Reflection and Positive Action

1. **Cardiovascular Conditioning and Muscle Toning**: How might the cardiovascular conditioning and muscle toning offered by *Splash*Dance improve your physical health and daily energy levels?

2. **Stress-Reducing and Mood-Enhancing Benefits**: In what ways could the stress-reducing and mood-enhancing benefits of *Splash*Dance impact your daily life and mental well-being?

3. **Cognitive Gains**: What cognitive gains do you hope to achieve through the rhythmic and fluid movements of *Splash*Dance, such as increased oxygen flow to the brain and improved neuroplasticity?

4. **Enhancing Flow**: Consider the barriers that prevent you from entering a state of flow. What are one or two specific actions you can take to minimize these distractions or challenges, thereby improving your ability to achieve and maintain flow during your training, and in your life?

5. **Understanding Flow**: Reflect on a time when you experienced a state of flow—where you were completely absorbed and lost track of time. What specific elements helped you achieve this state? How can you incorporate these elements more to prime flow more often?

CHAPTER 4

Riding the Waves to Well-Being – How Water Positively Transforms Us

The water is your friend. You don't have to fight with water; just share the same spirit, and water will help you move.

– Aleksandr Popov, Physicist and Engineer

The Essence of Aqua Fitness Water is a supportive, healing, and energizing environment that can enhance your health and vitality. Its unique properties make aquatic exercise a liberating experience, allowing you to feel uninhibited, flexible, and passionate. Submerged in chest height water, you may experience a sense of freedom, feeling less self-conscious and more open to engaging in physical activity.

Historical Waters: The Journey of Aquatic Exercise Water's relationship with health is ancient and awesome:

- **2400 BC**: Immersion in water was both a religious and healing practice.

- **1500 BC**: Early uses of water to reduce fever.

- **800 BC**: Healing waters in Bath, England, come into prominence.

- **Ancient Greece and Rome**: Water therapies for conditions like arthritic joints.

- **1700s**: Sigmund Hahn, a German doctor, pioneers hydrotherapy.

- **1980s**: First Aqua Dynamics presentations IDEA Health and Fitness World Congress

Fun Fact and Modern Waves: The Rise of Water Aerobics

Jack LaLanne, a renowned fitness professional, revolutionized aqua fitness in America. From opening his first spa in 1931 to innovating water aerobics in the 1950s, he utilized the buoyancy of water to relieve gravity's stress on the body. The popularity of water aerobics soared in the 1980s, marking a significant development in community fitness.

The Science of *Splash*Dance: Current Research and Benefits Contemporary studies highlight the extensive benefits of aquatic exercise:

- Enhanced injury prevention and recovery.
- Increased calorie burn compared to land-based exercises.
- Boosted metabolism and improved cardiovascular health.
- Greater flexibility and symmetrical muscle strengthening.
- Effective combat against the aging process through gentle yet effective resistance training.

Why is Water Such A Great Place to Train?

The Joy of Movement in Water Water's resistance is twelve times greater than air, providing a uniquely effective environment for fitness. Here are more reasons:

Proprioception: Because you're in the water and not on terra firma, you can reorient your body's proprioception. Proprioception is simply knowing, and feeling, your body's position in space. In water, your body learns to reorient its sense of position and movement, enhancing your coordination and spatial awareness.

Omnidirectional Resistance: Your body has the ability to move freely while suspended in the water, yet there is resistance in every direction you move it. For example, the faster you move your body parts, the more resistance you'll create, and the omnidirectional resistance is infinitely adjustable. You can slowly increase the range of motion to your joints and the resistance to your muscles to improve your strength and flexibility.

Cue the Conditioning and Toning Effects: To add to your conditioning, take advantage of the extra resistance that water offers. You can actively push and pull against it, adding speed, force, and leverage. The most effective way to *Splash*dance is to have your legs and arms exercising under the surface of the water. The result is a workout that feels refreshing and exhilarating.

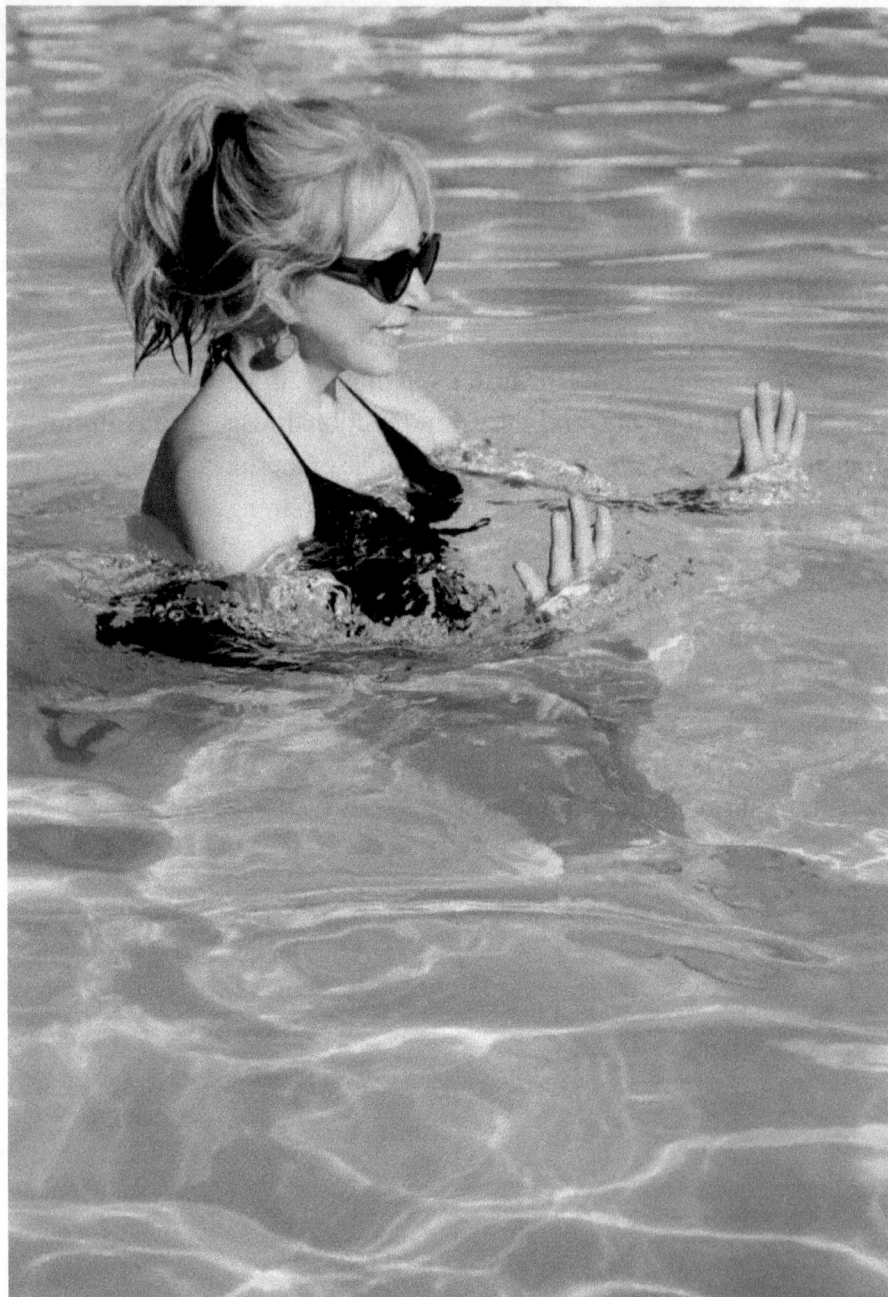

Photo: Lianna Tarantin

More Benefits of the *Splash*Dance Program

*Splash*Dance delivers a comprehensive fitness experience:

- **Muscle Conditioning Without Equipment**: The resistance provided by water means every movement helps to condition and balance muscle groups without the need for weights or machines.

- **Reduced Impact, Increased Buoyancy**: Water decreases the impact of exercises, reducing stress on joints and allowing for longer, more comfortable workouts.

- **Thermal Regulation**: Water naturally cools the body, preventing overheating and allowing for more extended, refreshing exercise sessions.

- ***Splash*Dance is a Complete Training**: *Splash*Dance offers the opportunity to work every cell of your body from your head to your toes. Train your brain, executive function, and learning systems with the cardiovascular or aerobic training, tone your muscles, shape up your mood, gain greater agility, balance, and flexibility, all beneficial and necessary for our fitness and well-being.

- **Social Fitness Matters**: In a group fitness training experience, you will get to meet people, have fun, and enjoy greater sociability.

- **A Fluid Path to Wellness** *Splash*Dance is more than just an aquatic exercise; it's a celebration of movement and health, tailored to meet the needs of an increasingly diverse fitness demographic. As society evolves, so too does the approach to wellness, and aqua fitness, particularly *Splash*Dance, stands at the forefront of this transformation, inviting you to dive in and experience the joy of getting wet.

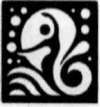

Questions for Reflection and Positive Action

- **Freedom in Water**: How does the sense of freedom you experience in water influence your feelings of lightness and discovery?

- **Unique Properties of Water**: How might the unique properties of water, such as increased calorie burn and improved cardiovascular health, motivate you to incorporate aquatic exercises into your repertoire?

- **Proprioceptive Feedback and Resistance**: In what ways does the proprioceptive feedback and omnidirectional resistance provided by water improve your physical fitness, particularly in terms of coordination and strength?

- **Reduced Impact and Buoyancy**: Given the reduced impact and increased buoyancy of water workouts, how could *Splash*Dance be particularly beneficial if you are recovering from an injury or managing chronic joint issues?

CHAPTER 5

The Science and Symphony of Aqua Dynamics

"We forget that the water cycle and the life cycle are one."

— Jacques Yves Cousteau, French naval officer, oceanographer, filmmaker, author, and inventor of SCUBA.

In this chapter, we dive into the vibrant essence of *Splash*Dance, exploring the intricate biomechanics, unique resistance properties and the pure exhilaration of movement that define this program. Here's what you will learn:

Enhance Your Fitness: Improve your aerobic endurance, muscular strength, flexibility, balance, agility, and social fitness.

Optimize Your Environment: Discover ways to harness the power of water to maximize fitness gains and happiness.

Elevate Your Experience: Integrate eclectic music and positive emotions to enhance your *Splash*Dance sessions.

The Science and Symphony of *Splash*Dance utilizes the unique properties of water to transform each session into a dynamic, fluid experience that enhances cardiorespiratory health, strengthens muscles, and boosts endurance, all within a fun and safe environment. Experience the joy of moving gracefully and powerfully, motivated by uplifting tunes that turn each training session into a celebration.

Biomechanics and Best Practices

*Splash*Dance offers a comprehensive and safe approach to aquatic fitness. Our guide includes a vast array of exercises, techniques, and strategies designed to optimize your movements for maximum health benefits, applying the best practices of biomechanics.

*Splash*Dance for Everyone: Variety and Inclusion

*Splash*Dance ensures no one is left behind. Our inclusive philosophy welcomes individuals of all abilities into a warm, caring, and respectful community. Celebrating diversity, the program shows how aquatic fitness benefits people of all ages, shapes, and physical capabilities.

Powerful Potential

Though gentle on the joints, *Splash*Dance effectively promotes bone health and offers a comprehensive, exhilarating fitness regimen that focuses on developing aerobic endurance, muscular strength, and flexibility.

Building Social Connections

More than just a physical workout, *Splash*Dance fosters a sense of belonging and community in a group setting. It is an effective antidote to loneliness, enhancing social connectivity and emotional well-being. Each session is a celebration of individual vitality and collective health, emphasizing the joy of positive connections and community thriving.

Guidelines, Tips, and Best Practices

To ensure the best experience, our well-structured *Splash*Dance program includes several key components:

1. **Safety First:** Always prioritizes your safety and well-being. In a group, use the "buddy system.

2. **Effectiveness Through Comprehensive Design:**

   - Exercises cover all planes, muscle groups, and directions.

   - Targets commonly weaker areas like the posterior arms, upper back, abdominals, gluteals, hamstrings, and the anterior tibialis (shin area).

   - Enhances flexibility in dominant, often tighter muscle groups such as the pectorals, erector spinae, hip flexors, quadriceps, and gastrocnemius.

   - Maintains proper alignment of the back, pelvis, knees, feet, and shoulders.

   - Incorporates posture-focused routines, offering cues, imagery, and reminders.

   - Gradually increase range of motion to improve flexibility and mobility.

3. **Enjoyment:** Emphasizes fun in a fluid environment with music, movement, and the chance to build positive connections.

4. **Challenge:** Encourages trying new moves, fostering growth and continuous improvement.

5. **Musical Enhancement:** Uses eclectic and themed music to boost mood, energy, and engagement, while promoting motivation, relaxation, and rejuvenation. Consider using music that "moves you," reminds you of a special time in your life, or expressive music that you can feel.

Join the Movement: This chapter is an invitation to embrace a movement that values health, vitality, happiness, and community. Whether you are a swimmer, non-swimmer, athlete, rehabilitating, or simply seeking a fun way to stay active, *Splash*Dance welcomes you to the rhythm of the water—where every movement counts and every splash brings joy.

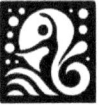

Questions for Reflection and Positive Action

Eclectic Music and Positive Emotions: How can uplifting music and positive emotions enhance your *Splash*Dance experience? What music moves you?

Biomechanics and Best Practices: What aspects of biomechanics and best practices can help optimize your movements and health benefits?

An Antidote to Loneliness: In what ways might *Splash*-Dance serve as an antidote to loneliness?

Inclusive Philosophy: How does the inclusive philosophy of *Splash*Dance resonate with your values or personal fitness goals?

CHAPTER 6

The *Splash*Dance Blueprint - Your Guide to Aquatic Success

Happiness comes in waves.

– Marlo Thomas, Actress, Producer, Author, Social Activist

*Splash*Dance isn't just about moving in the water; it's a structured program that targets all aspects of cardiovascular fitness, builds muscular strength and endurance, agility, balance, and flexibility. It's also a lot of fun! Ideally you will leave with a smile because aqua fitness tends to prime feelings of confidence, joy, and happiness.

Making the Most Of the Aqua Experience

To enhance your aqua exercise:

- Get comfortable in the pool. When you first enter the pool, continuously move your legs and arms to get and stay warm.

- Next find a water depth, preferably chest height, in which you can control your movements and not feel like you're floating away.

Each session can ideally last between 40 to 55 minutes and generally includes three key phases:

- **Thermal Warm-Up (5-10 minutes)**: This initial phase is designed to raise your body temperature and loosen your joints, setting the stage for more intense activity. It involves gentle movements that increase blood flow and prepare your muscles and joints for exercise.

- **Strength and Rhythmic Endurance Exercises (15-25 minutes)**: Dive into the heart of *Splash*Dance with a series of dynamic movements, like lunges or kicks, that challenge your major muscle groups, boost your cardiovascular health and strengthen you.

- **Cooldown (5-10 minutes)**: Wind down with stretches and gentle movements that help your body return to a resting state, reducing muscle soreness and enhancing relaxation.

Your Thermal Warm-Up for Thriving The thermal warmup is crucial for a successful *Splash*Dance session. Start with simple steps:

- Walk forward and backward for 15 steps each, swinging your arms to engage the whole body.

- Maintain good form: Keep your abdominals tight, shoulders relaxed, and head aligned with your spine. This posture ensures safety and maximizes the benefits of your workout. Gently lower your heels to the ground when water walking.

- Introduce variety: Try a variety of side-stepping, the grapevine movement, spins, and strides to keep things engaging and fun.

Breathing and Intensity Breathing is key in *Splash*Dance. Make sure you're not holding your breath as you move. Proper breathing not only keeps you energized but also ensures a steady flow of oxygen to your muscles. Use tools we will discuss, like the Borg scale or Talk Test, to monitor your exertion and adjust your pace accordingly.

*Splash*Dance 101: Quick Tips for Success Here are some practical tips to get the most out of your *Splash*Dance experience:

Water Depth: Depending on your comfort and goals, choose between waist-chest height shallow water and deeper water with a flotation device for non-impact training.

Comfort and Traction: Consider wearing some type of aqua shoes for added traction, resistance, safety, and comfort.

Prioritize Sun Protection: When you *Splash*Dancing, especially outdoors, be sure to safeguard your skin from harmful UV rays. Wearing a broad-spectrum sunblock with an SPF of at least 30-50, is essential. Reapplying sunblock every two hours, or more frequently if you are sweating or in the water, ensures continuous protection. Additionally, consider wearing protective clothing such as a rash guard and a wide-brimmed hat.

Drink Water: Hydration is crucial, particularly during physical activities. Drinking water helps regulate body temperature, lubricates joints, and delivers nutrients to cells, enhancing performance and recovery. The typical recommendation is to drink about 2-3 liters (.5 - .7 gallons) of water daily, but this requirement increases with physical activity due to sweat loss, which may go unnoticed in water. It's advised to drink at least 500 ml (about 17 ounces) of water around two hours before exercise to ensure adequate hydration. Additionally, take a few sips during your workout and drink sufficiently afterwards to replenish fluids lost during the activity.

Tips to Stay Warm in the Water

To keep your body temperature elevated to a comfortable level, and to avoid being too cold in the water, it's important to move continuously, using the large muscle groups of your body (your legs and arms). Wear a water fitness shirt, pants, like tights, and gloves. I wear water gloves for performance and to stay warm. I also wear a clean old pair of sneakers, or water shoes for extra warmth, protection, cushioning, for greater shock absorption, resistance, along with my tights and shirt. If you're cold or shivering, your muscles won't perform well. It's important to pay attention to how you feel, and what you might mindfully do to improve your FUNctional Fitness: that's around enjoyment and effectiveness of your training. And remember to keep moving.

Pool Temperature According to the Aquatics Exercise Association, the ideal temperature for the pool varies from 83-86 degrees Fahrenheit (28-30 degrees Celsius); this is the most comfortable temperature for most aqua fitness classes. This allows your body to react and respond normally to the onset of exercise, and the accompanying increase in body temperature prevents chilling or overheating.

If the water temperature is much higher or lower in either direction, you can make modifications accordingly. For very warm water, include lots more stretching and muscular conditioning, downplaying the cardiovascular aspects for safety's sake. In cold water, move! Increase your warmup time accordingly for safer stretching and better locomotion. Use direction changes, make whirlpools, reverse them, and explore the wide variety of aqua formations you will find herein.

Safety and Considerations While Vertical Aqua Fitness is safe and effective, always take precautions to ensure a secure environment:

Be mindful of your body alignment to prevent strain: Stand tall, keep your chin neutral, chest lifted, and engage your core.

Remember, the benefits of exercising far outweigh the risks associated with inactivity. You may, however, wish to discuss any new exercises with your healthcare provider if you have underlying health conditions.

Embrace the Splash Whether you're a fitness newbie or a seasoned athlete, *Splash*Dance offers a refreshing way to enhance your daily activities and overall well-being. Close your eyes and feel the water around you. Focus on your good form, listen to your body, and most importantly, have fun as you *Splash*Dance your way to health and vitality!

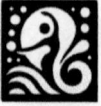

Questions for Reflection and Positive Action

Thermal Warm-Up Phase: How can the thermal warm-up phase of *Splash*Dance improve your readiness for more intense and frequent physical activity?

Strength and Rhythmic Endurance Exercises: Considering the strength and rhythmic endurance exercises in *Splash*Dance, what specific movements are you most excited to try?

Cooldown Phase: How does the cooldown phase contribute to your overall workout experience, and what stretches or movements do you find most beneficial for relaxation and muscle recovery?

Water Depth and Equipment Use: How does the choice of water depth and the use of equipment like water shoes and aqua gloves influence your comfort and performance in *Splash*Dance?

CHAPTER 7

Health in Every Splash - Unlock Your Potential

Vertical Aqua Fitness is an excellent exercise choice if you are looking for a low-impact, joint-friendly, enjoyable, and high benefit workout that offers a wide range of physical benefits. Whether you're aiming to fortify your cardiovascular fitness, build muscular strength and endurance, enhance flexibility, improve your balance, challenge your agility, train for a sport, or recover from an injury, *Splash*Dance is an awesome option to consider.

1. **Exercise Environment**: Vertical Aqua Fitness (VAF) is typically performed in shallow, or deeper water, either standing on the pool floor (shallow) or wearing a buoyancy belt, or using floatation devices (aqua barbells, noodles) to maintain an upright position in the deeper water. The water's buoyancy reduces the impact on joints and minimizes the risk of injury. In shallow water, the ideal depth is chest height, which allows you to experience buoyancy, reduce the impact forces, and yet control your body.

2. **Benefits**: Vertical Aqua Fitness offers numerous advantages, including cardiovascular conditioning, muscle toning, improved flexibility, and increased endurance. The water's resistance challenges the muscles and helps to build strength. It is also a great option for people with joint pain or limited mobility, as the water provides support and reduces stress on the joints. Further, a regular practice builds muscle, lowers blood pressure, and increases HDL (high density lipoproteins), good cholesterol.

3. **Aerobic Workout**: The exercises in Vertical Aqua Fitness involve various aerobic movements from different movement genres, such as jogging, jumping jacks, kicking, boxing, samba, and cross-country skiing motions. These activities elevate the heart rate, promoting cardiovascular fitness, toning, and calorie burning.

4. **Resistance Training:** The water's resistance makes every movement in Vertical Aqua Fitness more challenging. The resistance of the water provides constant engagement of the muscles, promoting toning and strengthening of the entire body. Movement underwater can create 12 times more resistance than movement on land. In addition, creating water currents and formations make changing directions, starting, or stopping movements a more challenging experience. Water barbells, resistance bands, and other aquatic equipment can be added for further resistance.

5. **Flexibility and Range of Motion**: The water's buoyancy assists in improving your flexibility and range of motion. Buoyancy reduces the effects of gravity and reduces stress on the joints. Further, the reduced gravity and support from the water allow you to move your joints through a wider range of motion without strain. Stretching exercises after your body is sufficiently warm in the water can enhance your overall flexibility. This is all based on your body's size, muscularity, and around the frequency, intensity, and duration of your training.

6. **Dimensions of Depth Forces**: In "shallow water," the depth plays an important and variable role. Training in water that is "nipple height," or at least above waist, is a safe bet. When you are up to your neck in water, you experience about 10% of your body weight (but be careful not to compromise your form). When you are chest high in the water, you are experiencing 25-35% of your

body weight, and when you are waist height, you can feel about 50% of your body weight. It's fun and smart to play around and experience training in different depths of water.

7. **Balance and Stability:** Water's natural buoyancy challenges balance and stability during exercises. Maintaining an upright position in the water requires core strength and coordination. These exercises help to improve balance and stability, which are essential for overall physical function and fall prevention.

8. **Rehabilitation and Injury Recovery:** Vertical Aqua Fitness is commonly used in rehabilitation programs due to its low-impact nature. The water's buoyancy and reduced stress on joints make it an ideal exercise option for individuals recovering from injuries or surgeries. It provides a safe and supportive environment for rebuilding strength and mobility.

9. **Social and Enjoyable:** VAF classes often create a social and supportive atmosphere. Group classes are popular, allowing you to exercise together while enjoying the benefits of water exercise. This can make the workout more enjoyable, increasing your motivation, adherence, and possible social ties.

10. **Suitable for Various Fitness Levels**: *Splash*Dance is inclusive; it's for people of ALL fitness levels and ages. The intensity of your workout can be adjusted by modifying your aquatic speed, range of motion, or by adding resistance. *Splash*Dance is excellent for novice exercisers, senior adults, pregnant women, and as an adaptive or rehabilitative exercise form. Additionally, it's a perfect complement for athletes looking to cross-train in an effectively powerful, yet gentle liquid environment.

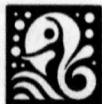

Questions for Reflection and Positive Action

1. **Cardiovascular Benefits**: With the cardiovascular benefits outlined, like improved heart health, how do you think regular *Splash*Dance sessions might impact your present, and longer-term health goals?

2. **Resistance Training**: Reflect on the resistance training aspects of *Splash*Dance. How does the concept of water providing 12 times more resistance than air influence your perception of its effectiveness in strength training?

3. **Flexibility and Range of Motion**: How might improving your flexibility and range of motion through *Splash*Dance affect other areas of your life, such as other activities of daily living.

4. **Adaptable Fitness Levels**: Given that *Splash*Dance can be adapted for various fitness levels, how do you see it fitting into your current or future fitness plans, especially as your needs, goals, and abilities evolve?

CHAPTER 8

Riding the Wave of Benefits to Whole Well-Being –A Holistic Approach

"The water is a miraculous substance that cures, calms, and cleanses."

- Jacques Yves Cousteau, Oceanographer, Inventor, Author

Introduction to the Benefits of *Splash*Dance

In this chapter, we examine how *Splash*Dance not only enhances physical health but also nourishes psychological resilience and brain health, all while aligning with the principles of lifestyle medicine. Here, you'll discover how each *Splash*Dance session contributes to a holistic improvement in physical robustness, mental clarity, emotional well-being, and overall lifestyle, making every splash a step towards a more fulfilled and healthy life.

1. More Physical Benefits of *Splash*Dance

- **Exercise Environment:** *Splash*Dance is adaptable to both shallow and deep-water environments, utilizing the natural buoyancy of water to reduce joint impact and allow for a range of exercises from simple movements to intensive workouts. Unlike swimming, you are vertical so your head, hair and face can stay dry.

- **Comprehensive Physical Advantages:** As we have discussed, you can achieve improved cardiovascular health, muscle toning, enhanced flexibility, and increased endurance. The resistance of water makes every movement a strength exercise, albeit with minimal risk to joints.

- **Dynamic Workouts:** From aerobic routines like jogging and jumping jacks to resistance training, each session is designed to elevate your working heart rate, boost your energy, lower distress, and promote calorie burning.

- **Flexibility and Mobility:** Water's buoyancy supports your body, allowing for a greater range of motion and helping with flexibility. This is particularly beneficial in rehabilitation settings where gentle movements are necessary and support challenging athletic performance.

- **Balance and Stability:** Water challenges your stability, requiring you to engage your core and improve overall coordination, essential for preventing falls and enhancing daily activities.

- **Accessibility:** Whether you're a beginner, rehabilitating, or someone with physical challenges, its adaptable nature, makes *Splash*-Dance suitable for all people.

2. Psychological Benefits of *Splash*Dance

- **Stress Management and Improved Mood:** The soothing effects of water combined with the endorphin release from exercise help significantly lower stress levels and enhance overall mood.

- **Mental Relaxation and Escape:** The rhythmic movements in water offer a mental break from daily stressors, promoting relaxation and a sense of well-being.

- **Enhanced Self-Esteem and Body Image:** The supportive nature of water workouts, along with the inclusive environment of group classes, boosts self-esteem and promotes a positive body image.

- **Social Interaction:** Group settings foster a sense of community and provide opportunities for social engagement, which can be motivational and emotionally uplifting.

3. The Brain Benefits of *Splash*Dance

- **Increased Brain Function:** Aerobic water exercises improve circulation, including to the brain, which enhances cognitive processes such as executive function, memory and problem-solving.

- **Neuroplasticity and Mental Health:** Regular physical activity like *Splash*Dance promotes neuroplasticity, aiding in the brain's ability to adapt and learn. Additionally, the positive emotions experienced during workouts contribute to better mental health.

- **Coordination and Multisensory Engagement:** Executing coordinated movements in water challenges the brain, enhancing focus and cognitive agility. The multisensory environment of water also stimulates neural pathways, boosting overall brain function.

- **Your Brain on Aerobic Exercise:** Research shows that when we exercise, our brains immediately light up with increased neurotransmitter levels. Neurotransmitters are the chemical messengers of the brain. These neurotransmitters are directly linked to positive increases in mood, energy and focus – with an added decrease in stress and anxiety levels. Research further demonstrates that aerobic activity improves blood flow and oxygen to the brain, leading to better cognitive function, enhanced memory and mindful attention.

Lifestyle Medicine and *Splash*Dance: Move, Nourish, Manage, Meet, Sleep, & Play

Lifestyle medicine, advocates for a proactive approach: preventing, treating, and reversing disease by promoting essential healthy behaviors. According to the American College of Lifestyle Medicine (ACLM), this includes physical activity, stress management, nutritious eating, optimal sleep, moderation in substance and alcohol use, and enriching social connections.

*Splash*Dance aligns seamlessly with these principles by virtue of its emphasis on exercise, stress reduction, and social health. Through rhythmic aerobic movements and resistance exercises in water, *Splash*Dance delivers. It offers cardiovascular health, flexibility, balance, agility, and strength, with enjoyable, socially engaging, and playful activities that significantly contribute to emotional well-being. The fun, supportive group environment is key to building community, and vital for mental and physical health. It champions the value of play in enhancing joy and creativity, making it an integral part of the holistic health experience.

*Splash*Dance can promote a positive upward spiral of goodness. It encourages increased motivation for better sleep and rest, helps manage stress, and nurtures healthier eating habits and as your overall well-being improves.

Lifestyle Medicine, similar to *Blue Zones,* advocates a plant-rich Mediterranean diet, emphasizing mindful eating, a "plant slant," savoring food with gratitude, and appreciating the people involved in its preparation.

*Splash*Dance embraces lifestyle medicine and how it promotes positive health.

A Multifaceted Approach to Well-being *Splash*Dance is a comprehensive program that can enhance many aspects of your well-being. It's easy-to-follow, rhythmic nature is soulful and uplifting. *Splash*Dance offers a unique opportunity to improve your health holistically, making each session not just a workout but a pathway to a more vibrant, happy, healthy life.

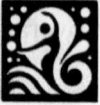

Questions for Reflection and Positive Action

1. **Psychological Benefits**: How might the psychological benefits of stress reduction and improved mood through *Splash*Dance influence your daily life?

2. **Brain Benefits**: In what ways could the valuable brain benefits of increased cognitive function and neuroplasticity affect your performance in other mental tasks?

3. **Balance and Stability Exercises**: Reflect on the role of balance and stability exercises in *Splash*Dance. How could improving these areas improve your overall well-being and functionality in daily activities?

4. **Holistic Approach**: *Splash*Dance encourages a holistic approach that values Lifestyle Medicine; which elements are most compelling to you and why?

CHAPTER 9

Aqua Dynamics in *Splash*Dance - Harnessing the Laws of Physics

You always find an answer in the sound of water.

- Zhuangzi

Understanding the Forces at Play *Splash*Dance isn't just a dance; it's a science. As you glide and power through the water, several key principles of physics optimize your workout, ensuring it is as effective as it is exhilarating.

- **Buoyancy**: Thanks to Archimedes' principle, your body is supported by the upward force of the water, which equals the weight of the water displaced. This buoyancy reduces the strain on your joints and allows you to perform movements that might feel impossible on land.

- **Resistance and Drag**: Moving through water means overcoming its natural resistance, caused by viscosity and density. This resistance is your friend in fitness, helping to tone and strengthen muscles more effectively than air resistance alone. Drag, the resistance that water exerts on your body as you move through it adds another layer, requiring you to exert more effort and thus enhancing your workout intensity.

- **Fluid Dynamics**: The flow of water around your body can be smooth (laminar) or chaotic (turbulent), each affecting your movement efficiency. By understanding these dynamics, you can optimize your movements to conserve energy and maximize your performance.

- **Newton's Laws of Motion:**

  - **First - Law of Inertia**: A body in motion stays in motion, and a body at rest stays at rest. In water, starting or stopping your movement requires overcoming inertia, demanding extra effort and energy, perfect for building strength.

  - **Second - Law of Acceleration:** The more force you apply, the greater your acceleration. The external forces produce a change in the velocity of the body in the direction of the force through the water, allowing you to adjust your workout intensity accordingly.

  - **Third - Law of Action and Reaction**: Every push or pull in water meets an equal counterforce, making every movement a potential muscle builder.

- **Eddy Resistance**: The swirling currents that form around your body and equipment create additional resistance. This so-called eddy resistance requires your muscles to work harder, delivering a more intense workout.

Leveraging Physics for Optimal Training Understanding and applying these physical laws can be enlightening and help you work, and play with the water, not against it, enabling more effective and enjoyable workouts.

- **Laws of Leverage**: Adjusting your body position, using equipment, or changing the depth at which you work alters the resistance you encounter. This manipulation of leverage can increase the difficulty of exercises or reduce it, depending on your needs.

- **Hydrostatic Pressure**: The deeper you go, the greater the pressure exerted by the water on your body, which has several beneficial effects:

  - **Circulatory Benefits**: Improves venous return and circulation, helping with swelling and delivering oxygen and nutrients more efficiently.

  - **Respiratory Enhancement**: Breathing against this pressure strengthens respiratory muscles, enhancing lung capacity.

  - **Postural Support**: The evenly distributed pressure helps align and stabilize your joints, reducing pain and supporting correct posture.

Aqua Physics at a Glance If you'd like to delve deeper into the physics of your movements in water, here are key concepts to consider:

- **Buoyancy**: Consider the concepts of buoyancy assisted, buoyancy supported, and buoyancy resisted to understand how different movements interact with the upward force.

  - **Buoyancy-Assisted Exercises: Exercises in which buoyancy helps to perform movements by reducing the body's effective weight.** An example is gentle leg lifts for someone with joint issues, where the water's lift aids in reducing strain on the joints while enabling movement.

- **Buoyancy Supported**: These exercises take advantage of buoyancy to support the body and reduce the impact on joints. For example, deep-water running where the water supports the body, reducing strain on the joints and spine while providing resistance to movement.

- **Buoyancy Resisted**: In contrast, these exercises use buoyancy as a form of resistance to make movements more challenging. An example is aqua jogging or walking against the natural lift of the water, where the legs must work harder to move through the water, thus providing a resistance workout.

- **Pressure**: Increases linearly with depth, optimizing circulation and muscle activation, especially in the lower body.

- **Drag**: Affected by your speed, the shape of your body, and how you move through the water, drag forces are a constant challenge enhancing your strength and conditioning.

By embracing these principles, you ensure your movements are safe, supported and that every mindful splash is a step toward greater health, strength, and vitality.

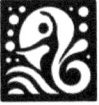

Questions for Reflection and Positive Action

1. **Principle of Buoyancy:** How does the buoyancy in the water influence your ability to perform exercises that might be difficult or impossible on land?

2. **Natural Resistance of Water**: Consider how the natural resistance of water can be used to your advantage in toning and strengthening muscles. How can that, and varying your speed and movement patterns, change your results?

3. **Newton's Third Law of Motion**: Reflect on how Newton's Third Law of Motion—action and reaction—applies to your movements in water. How can you apply this to enhance the effectiveness of your aqua fitness training?

4. **Increased Hydrostatic Pressure**: How might the increased hydrostatic pressure experienced at greater depths impact your physical health, especially in terms of circulatory and respiratory benefits?

CHAPTER 10

Fluid Forces - Mastering the 'Surface Area' Challenge in Water

Nothing is softer or more flexible than water, yet nothing can resist it.

- Lao Tzu, Chinese Philosopher, 571, BC

In the dynamic environment of *Splash*Dance, understanding how to optimize the surface area of your body and equipment can transform the resistance you encounter, the buoyancy you harness, and even the speed of your movements. Here's how mastering surface area can elevate your aqua fitness routine:

A Fluid Environment: Your Optimal Training Opportunity

1. **Enhancing Resistance Through Body Position:** The surface area of your body parts influences the resistance you encounter in the water. For example, expanding your arms during arm circles or extending your legs during kicks increases their surface area, thereby increasing resistance and intensifying the workout. This adjustment not only challenges your muscles more robustly but also boosts your strength and endurance.

2. **Buoyancy and Stability:** Increasing your surface area can aid in maintaining buoyancy and improving balance. Spreading your limbs not only makes you more stable in the water, which is partic-

ularly beneficial during balance-focused exercises like yoga poses or one-legged stands.

3. **Using Equipment to Modify Intensity:** Aquatic tools such as resistance gloves, paddles, or fins enlarge the surface area of your hands or feet. This expansion alters the dynamics of your movements by adding resistance and improving propulsion, essential for targeted muscle training and enhancing overall propulsion in the water.

4. **Tailored Aquatic Therapy:** In therapeutic settings, adjusting surface area using equipment like flotation devices enables precise control over the level of support and resistance. This adaptability is a key for rehabilitation, allowing for safe, effective exercise tailored to individual needs.

Body Alignment in *Splash*Dance

Proper body alignment is crucial to maximize the benefits of manipulating surface area in aqua fitness:

- **Consistency in Motion:** Ensure your knees and toes align, controlling your movements smoothly without any jerky motions.

- **Postural Integrity:** Maintain your natural spinal curves, ensuring your ears align over your shoulders, and your shoulders align over your hips. This alignment stabilizes your center of gravity and buoyancy, enhancing your balance and effectiveness in the water.

- **Dynamic Stability:** The aquatic environment will challenge your balance with its currents. Engage your core which is the group of trunk and hip muscles that surround the spine, abdominal viscera and hip. Keep your spine neutral, and position your feet properly to navigate these challenges effectively.

A Balancing Act: Transitioning from land to water exercise requires adjustments. The water's currents will push and pull, so contracting your trunk muscles and maintaining a strong, aligned posture is important as you increase the intensity of your movements.

Physical Fitness Spectrum in *Splash*Dance

Incorporating adjustments to surface area into your *Splash*Dance routine impacts various aspects of physical fitness: Aerobic Endurance, Muscular Strength, Muscular Endurance, Flexibility, Balance, Agility, and Coordination.

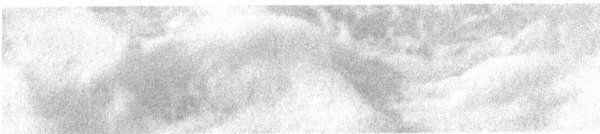

Physical Fitness Components

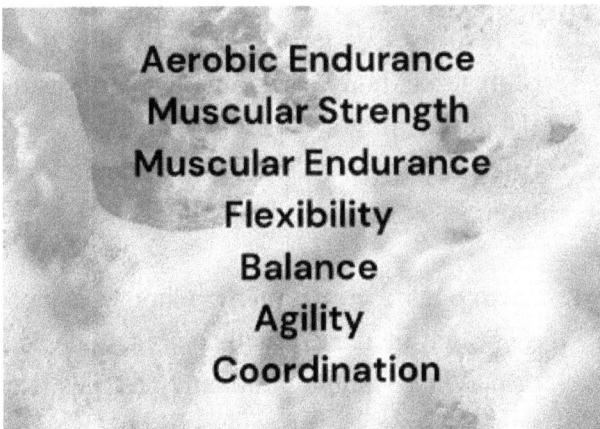

Aerobic Endurance
Muscular Strength
Muscular Endurance
Flexibility
Balance
Agility
Coordination

How you manage the surface area in your movements and any equipment you may use can enhance each fitness element. This chapter encourages you to harness the transformative effects of water through strategic surface area manipulation, ensuring every *Splash*Dance session is as effective as it is exhilarating.

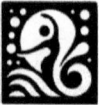

Questions for Reflection and Positive Action

1. **Manipulating Surface Area**: How does manipulating the surface area during your workouts make a noticeable difference in the resistance you feel in the water and in your training intensity?

2. **Proper Body Alignment and Posture**: In what ways has focusing on proper body alignment and posture during your water exercises influenced your overall fitness experience?

3. **Experiment with Surface Area**: During your next aqua fitness session, consciously alter the surface area of different body parts during exercises. For instance, try performing arm circles, varying arm positions or using different leg extensions during kicks to change the resistance. How does it feel?

4. **Incorporate Equipment**: Choose a piece of equipment that increases surface area, such as aqua gloves or paddles. Can you note any changes in the intensity and effectiveness of your workout?

5. **Focus on Alignment**: During your next session, pay special attention to your posture and alignment. Practice exercises like deep-water running or high knee walking, emphasizing keeping your spine aligned and vertical, ears over shoulders, and shoulders over hips. Observe any changes in your stability and core engagement.

6. **Track Changes**: Keep a journal of your observations when experimenting with different surface areas and equipment. Note any changes in your endurance, strength, balance, or comfort levels during workouts.

CHAPTER 11

Bounding - You Control the Impact Forces, Master Levels I, II, & III

Managing your impact awareness, or potential foot strike, is invaluable while exercising. A certain amount of impact is good for building bone density, but too much impact is harmful to the joints and body's structures. In *Splash*Dance, where the goal is to achieve effective training without undue stress on the body, here are some ideas to control the situation. Your manipulation significantly enhances your aqua training's intensity and effectiveness:

Bounding versus Non-Bounding Moves While aquatic striding movements like walking or running incur some joint stress during weight transition from one foot to the other, they have much less impact than similar moves on land. We can adjust the impact based on how we execute the movement. Bounding (impact), where both feet are off the pool bottom at some point and typically land with a toe strike (jogging), contrasts with non-bounding (low impact), where one foot always remains in contact with the pool bottom and typically lands with a heel strike (walking). Be sure to follow through with the movement after the initial contact with the pool bottom—heel, ball of the foot, toes, release—or toes, ball of the foot, heel, release.

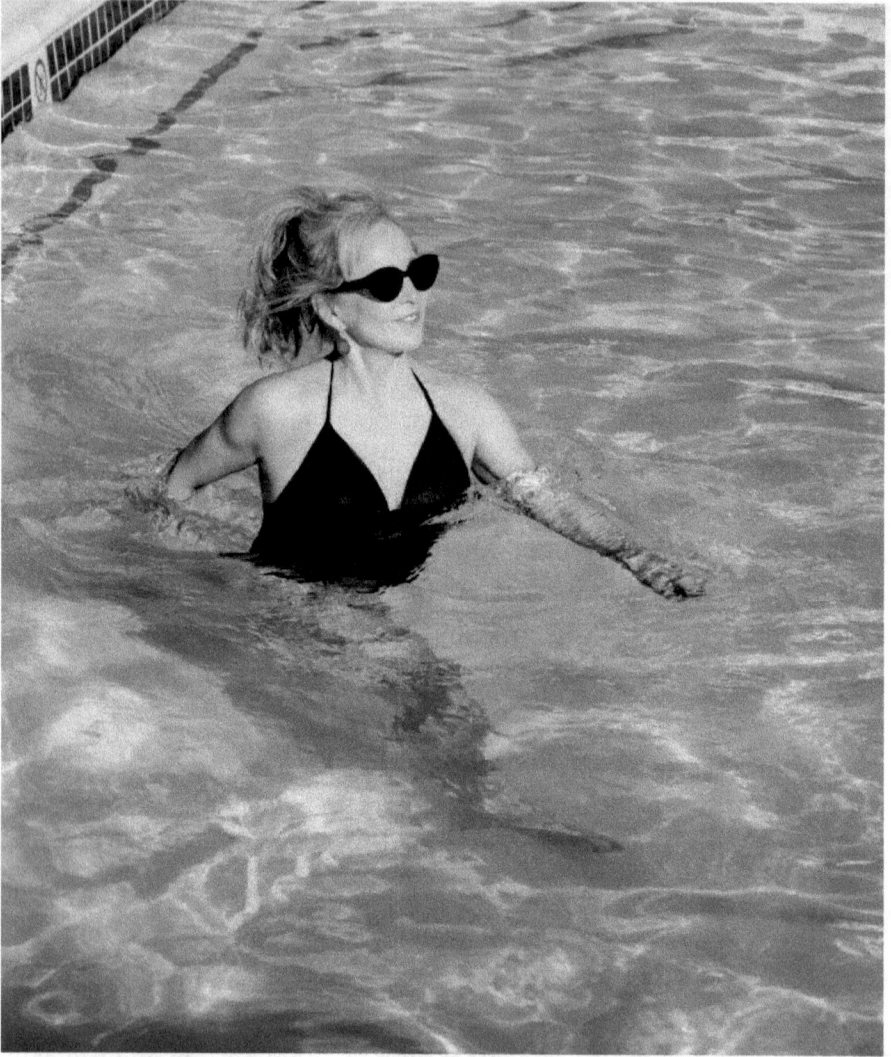

Photo: Lianna Tarantin

Modifying Impact: The impact level can also be modified by how we position the body in the water during our traditional aerobic choreography. An innovative program called Aquatics outlines three levels of intensity:

- **Level I:** Standing upright while propelling the body through the water with the legs as the primary source of power.

- **Level II:** Lowering the shoulders to the water's surface by flexing at the knee and hip joints, which involves the upper body more in propulsion.

- **Level III:** Keep both feet elevated from the pool bottom for more than one count at a time, using the upper body to maintain this suspended position. Level III movements can be interspersed throughout the workout for variety and challenge.

Intensity Is Different from Impact It's important to note that intensity and impact are not directly proportional. High-intensity movements can be non-impact, such as Level III aqua cross-country skiing.

Ways to Monitor Intensity During Aqua Fitness training, like in *Splash*Dance, intensity can be adjusted through several methods, depending on the specific movement:

- **Speed:** Increasing the speed of movement raises intensity, though it may decrease the range of motion.

- **Water Depth:** Moving from waist to armpit depth increases the difficulty due to more water displacement; however, too deep makes us too buoyant to maintain proper contact with the pool bottom and can compromise your control.

- **Length of Resistance (Lever):** For example, changing from a knee lift to a front kick with an extended leg increases the intensity by increasing the workload (the amount of water moved through).

- **Frontal Surface Area:** Increasing the area of the surface moving through the water increases resistance, such as jogging forward and dragging the arms slightly away from the body.

- **Force Application:** The more force applied to a movement, the greater the intensity.

- **More About Eddy:** Making movements less streamlined increases drag forces, which refers to the natural resistance that water exerts on a body moving through it. As you move your body parts through the water, the drag forces you to exert more effort, which helps strengthen muscles, improve endurance, and enhance cardiovascular fitness without the harsh impact associated with similar movements performed on land.

- **Changing Direction:** It requires more energy to change direction (overcoming inertia) than to continue in a straight line.

- **Arm Movements:** Arm patterns that resist the direction of travel can significantly affect the intensity of the overall movement. For example, jumping backward is intensified by performing breaststroke arm movements.

By understanding and applying these principles, you can increase the challenge and effectiveness of your training while minimizing unnecessary extra impact, ensuring a healthy, enjoyable, and sustainable fitness regimen.

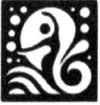

Questions for Reflection and Positive Action

1. **Bounding vs. Non-Bounding Movements**: How has understanding the difference between bounding and non-bounding movements changed your perception of the impact associated with different types of water exercises?

2. **Levels of Intensity**: Considering the three levels of intensity described (Levels I, II, and III), how do you think varying these levels can affect your progress?

3. **Exercise Implementation**: With what specific exercises might switch between bounding and non-bounding movements?

4. **Water Depth Variation**: Experiment with the different levels of water depth described. Note any differences in exercise difficulty and your personal comfort. What do you find most effective for your goals?

CHAPTER 12

Do the Locomotion With Me – Traveling in Rhythm

Locomotion in aqua fitness, often referred to as "traveling through the pool," encompasses a variety of dynamic movements aimed at propelling oneself through the water. This includes walking, jogging, running, jumping, and skipping—each offering different levels of intensity and engagement. In designing locomotion exercises, consider the pool's depth and layout. For varied experiences, create patterns that either maintain a consistent depth or transition from shallow to deeper water. In uniformly deep pools, navigate through lanes in inventive patterns such as sprinting up one lane and jogging back down another, effectively transforming the pool into an aquatic circuit. This approach not only enhances physical conditioning but also adds an element of fun and challenge to the workout.

Aqua Locomotion offers many great benefits:

Cardiovascular Fitness: Aqua Locomotion provides an effective cardiovascular workout. Moving against the resistance of the water requires more effort from the heart and lungs, resulting in increased working heart rate and improved cardiovascular endurance. Locomoting through the water can help strengthen your cardiovascular system, promoting better overall fitness.

Low-Impact Workout: The buoyancy of water reduces the strain on bones, joints, and connective tissues, making locomotion adaptable for those with joint issues, arthritis, or recovering from injuries. It allows for a safe and low-impact workout that minimizes the risk of injuries and joint discomfort.

Full-Body Workout: Locomotion engages multiple muscle groups throughout the body. Walking, jogging, or running in water requires the use of leg muscles, including the quadriceps, hamstrings, and calf muscles. Additionally, the resistance provided by the water engages the muscles of the core, arms, and shoulders as you maintain balance and stability during movement. This comprehensive engagement of muscles results in a full-body workout.

Not only do you enjoy body shaping and strengthening, but research also demonstrates that you build your bone as well, as in one study of post-menopausal women. The women, after a year of aqua fitness training, protected their bones, and had even slightly increased their spine's bone density.

Increased Resistance: The resistance of water is greater than air, providing a challenging environment for locomotion. Moving through the water requires more effort and energy expenditure compared to performing the same movements stationary, or on land. This increased resistance helps to build muscular strength, endurance, and power.

Balance and Stability: Water provides a dynamic and constantly shifting environment, challenging your balance and stability during locomotion. The need to stabilize and control your movements in response to the water's forces engages the core muscles and improves overall balance. This can be particularly beneficial for older adults or individuals seeking to enhance their balance and reduce the risk of falls. Water also provides a challenge for athletes training balance like soccer players or gymnasts

Variety and Fun: Locomotion, as in *Splash*Dance provides variety and a sense of fun. The sensation of traveling through water can be enjoyable and motivating.

Incorporating locomotion into your pool fitness program adds complexity and can enhance the overall benefits of your training. Whether you're walking, jogging, or performing more advanced, compound movements, locomotion in the water provides a low-impact, challenging, and enjoyable way to improve cardiovascular fitness, strength, balance, agility, and overall well-being. Locomotion is especially fun in a group, as you will see in the "Aqua Formations" section.

In a group, introducing moving formations such as "the snake" can leverage increased eddy drag for a more challenging workout, while formations like circles may increase resistance. Traveling across the pool and adding interactions such as swinging partners, meeting in the middle of the pool for a "do-si-do," sharing high-fives, or even initiating a playful basketball jump shot adds a delightful social element. Creating moving circuits, or games, like tag or relay races, can infuse more energy and laughter while cultivating friendly competition and camaraderie.

Incorporating locomotion and traveling exercises into a pool fitness program not only diversifies the workout experience but also significantly amplifies the health benefits, making it a fantastic, low-impact way to enhance cardiovascular fitness, strength, balance, and overall well-being. Experience the transformative power of aquatic locomotion—where every movement is a step towards a healthier you.

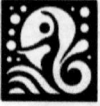

Questions for Reflection and Positive Action

1. **Benefits of Locomotion**: Which benefits of locomotion resonate most with you (e.g., cardiovascular fitness, low-impact workout, full-body exercise, increased resistance, balance and stability, variety, and fun) and why?

2. **Variety of Movements**: Out of the variety of movements described (like walking, jogging, jumping, skipping, frog kicks, scissor kicks), which aqua activities would you like to creatively incorporate into your next water workout?

3. **Social Interactions and Well-being**: How enjoyable do you think "locomoting," or creating aqua formations with others would be?

CHAPTER 13

Aqua Resistance, Persistence and Levers - Get Fit Without Gear

You can increase the intensity of your aqua training without using equipment by manipulating various factors. Here are some ways to do so:

1. **Speed and Tempo:** Increase the speed at which you perform your exercises in the water. Whether it's water running, or performing a dynamic *Splash*Dance aerobics circuit, moving faster requires more effort and increases your exercise intensity. You can also vary your tempo by incorporating interval training, alternating between high-intensity bursts and periods of active recovery.

2. **Range of Motion (ROM)**: Refers to the angular distance and direction a joint can move in a flexed and extended position. For example, when performing leg kicks or arm movements, try extending your limbs further or increasing the amplitude (height, in a jump), full extension, and distance) of your movements. This more intensely challenges your muscles and range of motion ROM capabilities.

3. **Resistance Techniques**: Increase the intensity by utilizing the water's resistance. Engage in movements that involve pushing, pulling, and moving against the water's resistance. Examples include water push-ups against the pool wall, "resisted" walking (adding

hands at your hips or out to the side to increase surface area), deep-water running, performing cross-country ski movements, or adding props.

4. **Vertical Movements**: Incorporate vertical movements in deep water to increase intensity. Activities like treading water, high knees running, jumping jacks, or scissor kicks engage multiple muscle groups and elevate your heart rate. These movements require continuous effort to stay afloat and provide a challenging, energizing, and empowering cardiovascular workout.

5. **Change of Direction**: Incorporate direction changes and patterns in your pool workout. Instead of moving, in shallow or deep water a straight line, incorporate lateral movements, zigzags, or circular patterns. Changing directions challenges different muscle groups and adds variety to your workout, increasing overall intensity and the fun factor.

6. **Interval Training**: Implement interval training principles in your pool workout. Alternate between periods of higher intensity and active recovery. For example, you can perform all-out sprints for a set time or distance, followed by stretching, and then a period of slower, relaxed movements. This interval approach allows you to work at a higher intensity while allowing for periods of rest and recovery.

7. **Incorporate Plyometric Exercises**: Plyometric exercises involve explosive movements that can be adapted to the pool. Examples include squat jumps, tuck jumps, or explosive arm movements in the water. These exercises engage fast-twitch muscle fibers, increase power, and elevate the intensity of your workout. Check out the "Athletic Performance and Priming Plyometrics" chapter.

Intensity and The Magic of Lever Lengths

In aqua fitness training, the concept of using long and shorter levers refers to manipulating the length of your limbs (arms and legs) or the distance between your joints to modify the intensity and resistance of the exercises. Here's an explanation of the difference between long and shorter levers and how to put this into action:

1. **Long Levers**: Long levers involve fully extending your limbs to increase the leverage and resistance in the water. By elongating your arms or legs, with extended alternating leg kicks forward, you effectively increase the surface area. This creates more resistance against the water. Increased resistance challenges the muscles involved in the movement, making the exercise more intense.

Here's an example: In aqua fitness, when you perform a bicep curl exercise, extending your arm fully by straightening it completely increases the length of the lever, creating more resistance as you bend your elbow against the water.

2. **Shorter Levers**: Shorter levers involve bending your joints to reduce the leverage, resistance, and intensity in the water. By decreasing the length of your limbs or the distance between your joints, you reduce the surface area and resistance encountered during the exercise, which can make the movement easier.

Example: When performing a leg kick exercise in water with bent knees instead of with your legs extended, it shortens the levers, lessening the resistance. Using long and shorter levers is beneficial in aqua fitness training for several reasons:

- **Progressive Intensity**: By adjusting the lever length, you can progressively increase or decrease the resistance encountered during exercises.

- **Targeting Specific Muscles:** Long levers engage larger muscle groups and require more effort, while shorter levers can isolate specific muscles or focus on smaller muscle groups.

- **Customization**: Different individuals have varying levels of strength and flexibility. Exercises can be customized to accommodate individual needs, abilities, and fitness goals by using long or shorter levers.

- **Variety and Progression**: Incorporating both long and shorter levers into aqua fitness routines adds variety and helps prevent plateauing. It allows you to continually challenge yourself and progress in your fitness journey.

When utilizing long and shorter levers in aqua fitness training, it's important to maintain proper form and technique to ensure safety and effectiveness. Focus your mindful attention on maintaining good alignment, engaging your core, and performing controlled movements (with a smile) throughout the exercises.

More About Lever Lengths

Using shorter levers and longer levers in aqua fitness training can offer different benefits due to the varying levels of intensity and muscle engagement. Here's a breakdown of the benefits associated with each:

Benefits of Using Shorter Levers:

1. **Increased Speed and Range of Motion**: Shorter levers require less effort to move through the water, allowing for faster movements and a wider range of motion. This leads to improved agility, coordination, and fluidity in your training.

2. **Muscle Isolation**: Shorter levers can target specific muscle groups with more precision. By reducing the leverage, you can isolate and focus on particular muscles, enhancing their strength and definition. This can be especially beneficial for rehabilitation, injury prevention, and muscle imbalances.

3. **Joint-Friendly**: Using shorter levers reduces the stress and impact on joints, making it a suitable option for individuals with joint issues or those recovering from injuries. The decreased lever length helps to minimize joint compression and excessive strain on the joints during movements, providing a low-impact workout.

4. **Flexibility Improvement:** You can improve your flexibility by bending your joints to create shorter levers. Shorter levers make it easier to achieve and maintain positions that challenge your flexibility.

Benefits of Using Longer Levers:

1. **Increased Resistance:** Longer levers generate more resistance against the water due to the larger surface area they create. This heightened resistance makes the exercises more challenging, requiring greater muscular effort and engagement. It helps to build strength and endurance throughout the body.

2. **Full-Body Engagement:** Longer levers engage multiple muscle groups simultaneously, promoting a full-body workout. The increased resistance activates a larger portion of your muscles, leading to improved muscular strengthening and toning.

3. **Cardiovascular Conditioning**: Working with longer levers in the water requires more effort and energy expenditure, resulting in an increased heart rate and improved cardiovascular fitness. It can help boost your endurance and contribute to a more efficient cardiovascular system.

4. **Calorie Burn**: The higher resistance encountered with longer levers leads to a greater calorie burn during aqua fitness session, and after. The increased effort required to move longer levers through water can support weight management.

It's important to note that the choice between using shorter levers and longer levers depends on individual fitness goals, abilities, and the specific exercise or movement being performed. You can incorporate a combination of both lever lengths into your aqua fitness program to provide variety, strengthen muscle groups, cross-train, and challenge yourself in different, engaging ways.

Remember to listen to your body, stay hydrated, and gradually increase, and vary the intensity of your aqua fitness training over time, trying different ways to move well.

Questions for Reflection and Positive Action

1. **Personal Reflection**: After trying the techniques described, such as speed and tempo or vertical movements, which method challenged you the most and why?

2. **Technique Improvement**: How can adjusting your range of motion or changing the direction of your movements impact your workout intensity? Try these during your next session and note any differences to how you feel.

3. **Community Engagement**: Discuss and share with other aqua enthusiasts how you can customize your training using long and short levers. What are some unique variations and how have these techniques helped your fitness progress?

CHAPTER 14

Complete Thermal Warmup Wisdom - Preparing to *Splash*Dance

A thorough warm-up is essential to prepare your body for the dynamic movements that are about to follow. To maximize your safety and boost your performance, here's how to effectively achieve a **Comprehensive Thermal Warm-up:**

- **Initiate with a Slow Jog**: Begin your session with a slow 30-45-second jog or easy locomotion to gently raise your core temperature and loosen the muscles. This initial activity sets the stage for increased blood flow and energy production.

- **Dynamic Leg Movements**: Follow with dynamic leg movements:

  - To enhance leg muscle elasticity and readiness, open and close your legs doing easy jumping jacks for 30 seconds, lowering heels to the pool floor. Hands on hips.

  - Perform a slow, controlled jump from front to back with feet together for another 30 seconds, focusing on coordination and light impact.

Muscle Activation:

Bring each knee to the chest alternately for 30 seconds, jogging lightly to increase hip flexibility and prepare your legs for more vigorous activities.

Point and flex your feet to improve ankle mobility and your readiness for water resistance movements.

Integrate Walking and Striding: Throughout your warmup and cooldown, include water walking and easy striding to help maintain warmth and muscle engagement.

Physiological Benefits of a Warmup:

Increases Core Temperature: A gradual warm-up can raise muscle temperature by up to four degrees Fahrenheit, enhancing calorie burning and energy efficiency.

Prevents Injuries: It serves as an ideal transition, increasing the elasticity of muscles and connective tissues, thus preparing them for the physical challenges ahead.

Enhances Muscle Contraction and Efficiency: Warm muscles contract faster and with greater force, allowing for more effective movements.

Improves Circulation and Waste Removal: Enhanced blood flow ensures that working muscles receive ample oxygen and nutrients and helps in quicker removal of waste products and carbon dioxide.

Speeds Up Nerve Messages: Faster nerve responses improve reaction times and coordination during your *Splash*Dance routine.

Concluding the Warmup: As you end your warm-up session, revisit lighter activities like gentle striding or water walking before transitioning into your final stretches. This helps in reducing post-exercise fatigue and optimizes recovery.

Have fun warming up and get physically and mentally ready for the exhilerating activities that follow.

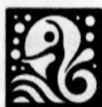

Questions for Reflection and Positive Action

1. **Reflect on the Importance of Warmup:** How has your perception of warming up changed after learning about its physiological benefits?

2. **Evaluate Your Current Warmup Routine:** Before performing your next physical activity, what's your warmup plan? Are there specific techniques you might enjoy?

3. **Commit to Consistency:** Consider setting reminders, preparing a set playlist of warmup music, or partnering with an accountability buddy to ensure you are training consistently and safely, including with a proper warmup.

CHAPTER 15

The Magic of Performing Water Walking and Aqua Striding

Transform walking in the water into a superb total-body workout that is gentle on your joints, easy on your back, and refreshingly energizing.

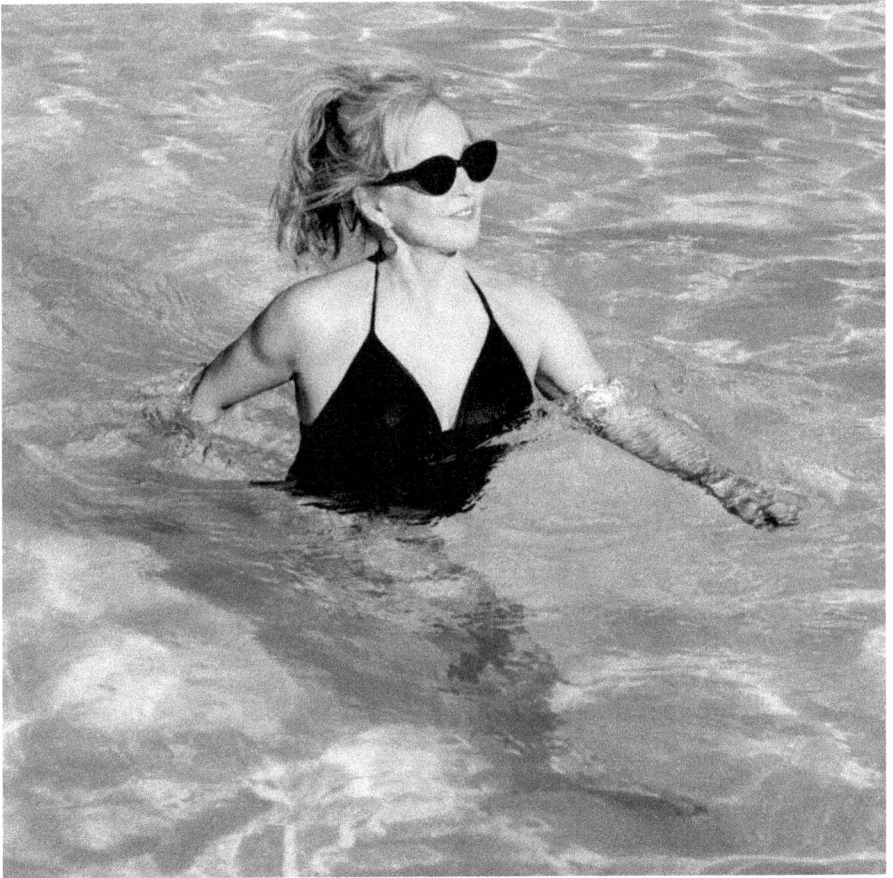

Photo: Lianna Tarantin

Water Walk in water that's waist or chest deep, and:

1. **Find an Appropriate Location:** Choose a shallow body of water with enough space to allow comfortable movement. Again, a waist or chest height ensures optimal buoyancy, comfort, and control.

2. **Warm-up:** Warm up your body on land to prepare your muscles, focusing on areas that will be actively engaged during the water walking, then stretch.

3. **Enter the Water:** Gradually walk into the water until you reach the desired depth, allowing your body to acclimate to the temperature and buoyancy.

4. **Start Walking:** Lift your legs and move them forward as if you were walking on land. It's important to ensure you maintain an upright posture and engage your core to stabilize your body against the natural resistance of the water. Vary your arm movements.

5. **Control Your Movements:** Maintain a controlled, steady pace, adjusting between walking and jogging based on your fitness goals. Pay attention to maintaining good form to maximize the benefits and prevent strain.

6. **Increase Intensity:** Amp up the challenge by walking faster, extending your training duration, or incorporating moves like side steps, high knees, and locomoting, (or traveling across the pool) to enhance your cardiovascular and muscular engagement.

7. **Walk in Rhythm:** Boost your motivation and enjoyment by creating a playlist that moves you.

Benefits of Water Walking:

1. **Low Impact:** The buoyancy of water significantly reduces the impact on joints especially compared to land exercises; it's ideal for those with joint pain or recovering from injuries.

2. **Cardiovascular Fitness:** Water walking increases heart rate and improves endurance and stamina through continuous movement against water resistance.

3. **Muscle Toning and Strength:** Engages multiple muscle groups, including the core, legs, and arms, through the resistance provided by the water.

4. **Balance and Coordination:** Water's natural instability challenges your balance and coordination, enhancing these skills over time.

5. **Weight Management:** Acts as an effective calorie burner, aiding in weight management and promoting a healthy metabolism.

6. **Rehabilitation and Recovery:** Often incorporated into rehabilitation to support recovery from injuries or surgeries, it provides gentle yet effective training.

7. **Excellent Warm-up and Cool Down:** Primes muscles for the activities to come during training and after, luxuriously lubricates the joints, and feels great.

Variations of Water Walking:

1. **Forward Water Walking:** The basic form, focusing on maintaining an upright posture and engaged core while moving forward. Walk toe, ball, heel down.

2. **Backward Water Walking:** Walk backward to target different muscle groups, enhance coordination, and build proprioception, your body's awareness in space.

3. **Sideways Water Walking:** Engage inner and outer thigh muscles by taking side steps, alternating directions to add variety.

4. **High-Knee Water Walking:** Lift your knees higher than usual to intensify the workout, engaging the hip flexors and core muscles more effectively.

5. **Heel-to-Toe Water Walking:** With each step, reach the heel to the toe of the opposite foot to challenge balance and coordination.

6. **Cross-Country Water Walking:** Mimic cross-country skiing or hiking movements by moving in a zigzag or serpentine pattern, adding complexity and fun to the routine.

7. **Interval Water Walking:** Alternate between periods of easy pacing and bursts of increased speed or intensity to boost cardiovascular health and calorie burn.

8. **Water Walking with Resistance Equipment:** Utilize water barbells, resistance bands, or ankle weights to enhance strength, endurance, and for a challenge.

More Water Walking and Striding Moves

1. **Walk/Jog Lifting Knees High & In Front**: Walk or jog through the water, lifting your knees as high as possible directly in front of you, engaging the lower insertion of your abdominals and your hip flexors.

2. **Walk/Jog Lifting Knees Up, Hips Externally Rotated**: While moving forward, lift your knees outward in a rotated fashion from the hip, enhancing the engagement of the outer thigh and gluteal muscles.

3. **Walk/Jog Lifting Heels Toward Buttocks (hamstring curls)**: Walk or jog forward and backward, bringing your heels up toward your buttocks, effectively working your hamstrings.

4. **Walk/Jog Lifting Feet in Front, Hips Externally Rotated**: As you walk or jog, lift your feet up in front of you with hips externally rotated, mimicking a motion of trying to reach toward your ankle in front of you, targeting the inner thighs and hip flexors.

5. **Step Kick Front (Hip Flexion/Knee Extension)**: Take a step, then kick the same leg forward, keeping the knee extended; it works the hip flexors and quadriceps.

6. **Step Kick and Hamstring Curl (Hip Extension/Knee Flexion)**: Step forward, kick one leg back, and then curl the heel towards the buttocks, targeting the glutes and hamstrings.

7. **Side Steps (Abduction/Adduction)**: Step side to side, moving your legs away from and towards your body, to work the muscles on the outer and inner thighs.

8. **Adductor Cross Over**: Cross one leg over the other as you step sideways; focus on your inner thigh muscles as you move your leg back to starting position.

9. **Inward Rotation Walks**: Walk with your toes pointing inward, rotating at the hips. This may feel funny, but it helps strengthen the muscles responsible for rotating the legs inward.

10. **Outward Rotation Walks**: Walk with your toes pointing outward, rotating at the hips, engaging, and strengthening the external rotators of the hip.

11. **DorsiFlexion Walks**: Walk with your toes pulled up towards your shin (dorsiflexed), focusing on engaging the shin muscles, which can help improve ankle stability, mobility, and your balance.

12. **Power striding**: Take long strides, flex your knees and hips as you step forward; straighten as your legs come together, hands at side swinging under the water)

Listen to your body's cues. Start at a pace and intensity that matches your fitness level. Gradually increase the duration, speed, intensity, and surface area as your fitness improves. Why not make water walking an enjoyable part of your exercise plan?

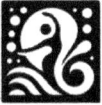

Questions for Reflection and Positive Action

1. **Water Walking for Low-Impact Fitness**: In what ways can water walking support your fitness goals including energization, strengthening, flexibility. agility, power, relaxation?

2. **Cardiovascular Benefits of Water Walking**: How might increasing your cardiovascular fitness though water walking improve your stamina, mood, and well-being?

3. **Variety in Water Walking**: Which water walking moves would you like to try or enjoy?

4. **Balance and Coordination**: How do you think practicing water walking could improve your balance and coordination?

5. **Social Aspects of Group Water Walking**: How could participating in *Splash*Dance impact your social well-being, adherence, and motivation to exercise?

CHAPTER 16

Going Deep - Dynamic Deep-Water Exercise Training

Deep-water exercise, a pivotal component of the *Splash*Dance program, harnesses the unique properties of water, offering a training modality that is gentle, powerful, and effective. Performed with the body fully suspended in water and supported by flotation devices like belts, noodles, or paddleboards, deep-water training can pack a powerful punch. Utilizing the water's neutral resistance properties and the depth forces, deeper water delivers an optimal training challenge and experience.

Deep water running and deep-water exercises evoke positive feelings and enjoyment. The buoyancy and support of the water create a sense of weightlessness, which can be incredibly liberating and stress-relieving. This sensation often leads to a heightened mood and a feeling of lightness, both physically and emotionally.

The natural resistance of the water provides a challenging yet gentle workout. Aqua fitness can boost your confidence and foster a sense of accomplishment, contributing to your overall emotional well-being. Deep water exercise, like in *Splash*Dance can also be a social and engaging activity, with opportunities for positive interaction and community building. The camaraderie and support from fellow participants can really enhance the experience. The combination of the fun and challenging deep-water activity, social connection, and the calming influence of water can leave you feeling energized and refreshed. This holistic blend of benefits makes deep water exercise not only effective but also highly enjoyable, and leave you wanting more.

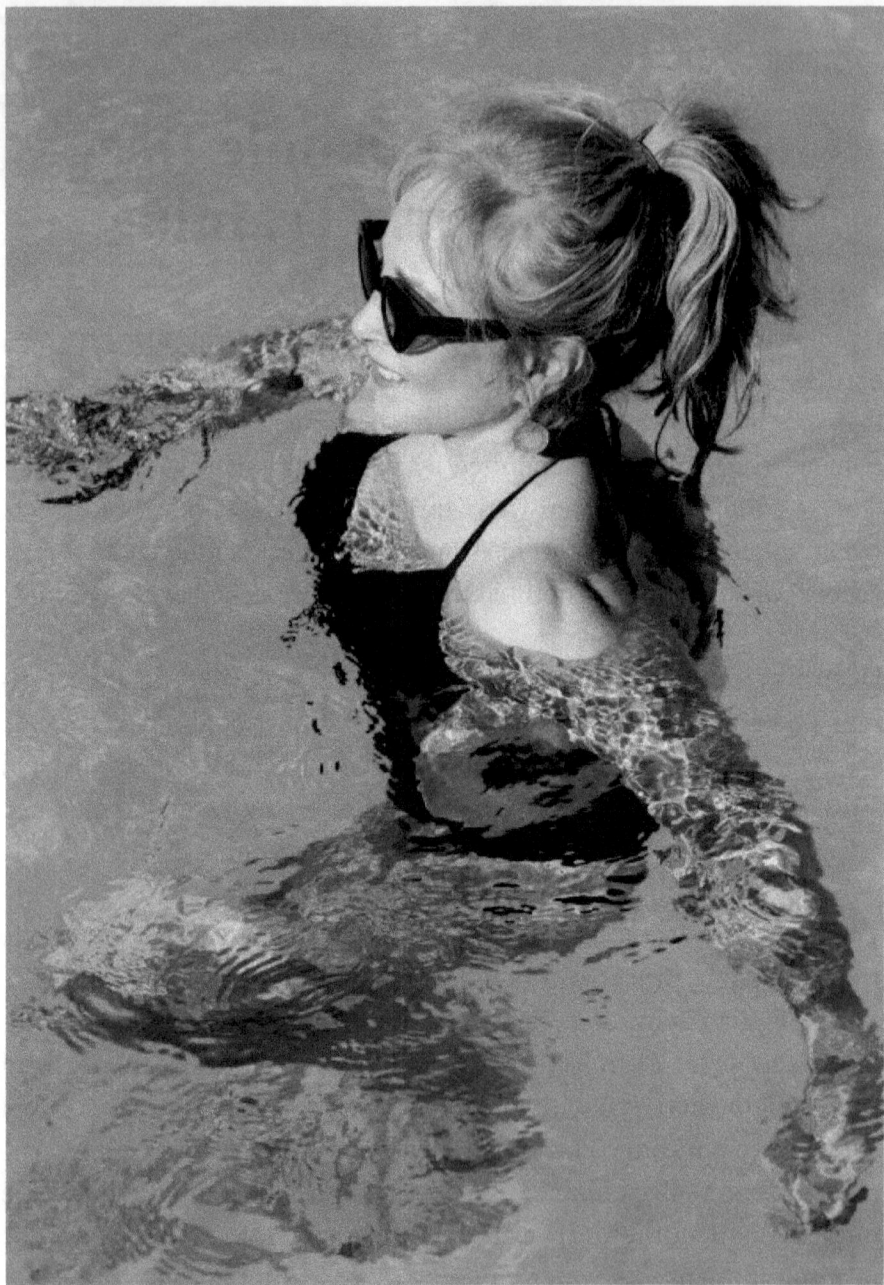

Photo: Lianna Tarantin

Why Choose Deep-Water Training?

- **Non-impact Environment:** Deep-water training provides a completely non-impact environment, where the buoyancy of water counteracts gravity's pull. This makes it ideal for everyone, from fitness beginners to athletes, offering a joint-friendly option for recovery and stress-free training.

- **Efficient Muscular Workout:** Submerged in water, both your upper and lower body confront constant resistance. Since water's resistance is 12 times greater than air, these conditions foster the simultaneous development of muscular endurance and aerobic capacity.

- **Enhanced Muscular Balance:** Unlike land workouts that are limited by gravity's downward pull, deep-water exercise offers multidirectional resistance. This promotes balanced muscle strength as movements in one direction are equally resisted in the opposite direction.

- **Improved Kinesthetic Awareness:** The absence of solid ground to stabilize movements challenges your balance and coordination in deep-water, strengthening stabilizing muscles and enhancing proprioception.

Deep-Water Running: A Core Activity Deep-water running, or aqua jogging, replicates land running movements in a fluid environment, offering cardiovascular benefits without the impact on joints. Here's more for you to get started:

- **Technique and Posture:** Begin with an upright posture, using flotation aids if needed. The goal is to maintain alignment while performing land running motions, driving knees up and using arms for balance and propulsion.

- **Variations for Increased Challenge:** Modify stride lengths, integrate interval training, or use resistance tools like aqua gloves to intensify the workout and target different muscle groups.

Deep-Water Training Techniques and Tips

- **Starting Off:** Use a buoyancy belt, or noodle, to effortlessly maintain an upright position, allowing you to focus on executing movements with precision.

- **Exercise Variations:** From jogging to high knees, jumping jacks, or cross-country ski movements, each variation targets specific aspects of physical fitness, such as endurance, strength, or agility.

- **Engagement and Enjoyment:** The enjoyable nature of moving in water, combined with the significant physical and mood benefits, provides motivation and adherence to the training.

Deep-Water Fun Facts and Challenges Variations and intensity adjustments in deep- water running can be tailored to increase workout challenges or focus on specific muscle groups. Techniques such as high knees, hamstring curls, or scissor kicks, not only engage different muscles but also enhance coordination.

Transformative Effects of Deep-Water Training

- **Physical Transformation:** Regular participation can significantly improve posture, increase flexibility, and strengthen muscles symmetrically.

- **Mental and Emotional Benefits:** The soothing effects of water make deep- water exercise both a physical and therapeutic activity, alleviating stress and enhancing overall well-being.

- **Accessibility:** Its gentle nature makes deep-water training suitable for those recovering from injuries, managing joint pain, or conditions like arthritis.

Deep-water training provides a challenging holistic workout that rejuvenates your mind and body. Whether you are recovering from an injury, looking to boost your athletic performance, or simply seeking a fun and effective way to stay active, *Splash*Dance deep-water training offers an incredible approach to meet these goals.

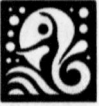

Questions for Reflection and Positive Action

1. **Non-Impact Environment of -Water Training**: How might the non-impact environment of deep-water training change your perspective on high-intensity workouts, especially if you have concerns about joint pain or injury recovery?

2. **Efficient Cardiovascular and Muscular Workout**: How can the powerful cardiovascular and strength training benefits enhance your fitness and your life?

3. **Improved Kinesthetic Awareness**: How can your improved kinesthetic awareness from deep-water exercise impact other areas of your life, including your balance, coordination, or daily physical activities?

4. **Enjoying Deep-Water Running**: What steps can you take to make deep-water running even more enjoyable and fun?

5. **Identifying Specific Deep-Water Exercises**: What are your favorite deep-water exercises and moves?

CHAPTER 17

Making Waves - Your *Splash*Dance Playbook and Moves Manual

Welcome to a refreshing journey through the dynamic realm of *Splash*-Dance. This chapter presents a curated list of aqua exercises and cool water fitness moves categorized by phase—thermal warm-up, aerobic activity, conditioning, and cooldown (with a separate Aqua Abdominals moves chapter). Each movement is detailed with an easy-to-follow description, for you to execute in the water's supportive environment.

Whether you're newly beginning your aquatic adventure or you're an experienced enthusiast honing your skills, or an athlete training for high performance, this guide offers a well-structured path to ensure a fulfilling, safe, effective workout experience. Delight in the exhila-rating world of *Splash*Dance, where the freedom and joy of movement harmoniously blends with the playful spirit of the water!

Thermal Warmup

Marching, Walking, Striding – To increase your body temperature and heart rate, march, walk, and stride with high knees, pumping arms back and forth for increased heart rate. Maintain your upper body posture, vary your arms with hands on hips, out to side, or train working your biceps and triceps. Vary your intensity for your desired outcome. Adding music that moves you is recommended.

Light Easy Jogging – pump your arms, and jog with knees up and then heels up.

Samba Marching with Spins - March with a rhythmic samba beat, moving your hips side to side and in circles, adding spins for fun, agility, balance, and a laugh.

Shake It Up, Shake It Down – To make the most of the water's magical properties, perform most movements with your arms and hands submerged. Loosen up by your shaking arms and legs gently in the water to relax muscles.

Water Walk and Tarzan – "Beat" your chest, tapping gently with fisted or flat hands, to reduce distress, boost your energy and vitality, decrease pain and cravings!. For a circulation boost, massage your kidneys gently.

Aerobic Exercise

1. **Jumping Jacks** - Perform traditional jumping jacks in the water. Start with your feet together and then jump to a hip wide stance while simultaneously bringing your arms from your side to the top of the water. Vary your speed, the surface area, and moves: Jumping Jack to the side, laterally with front raise, extended arms.

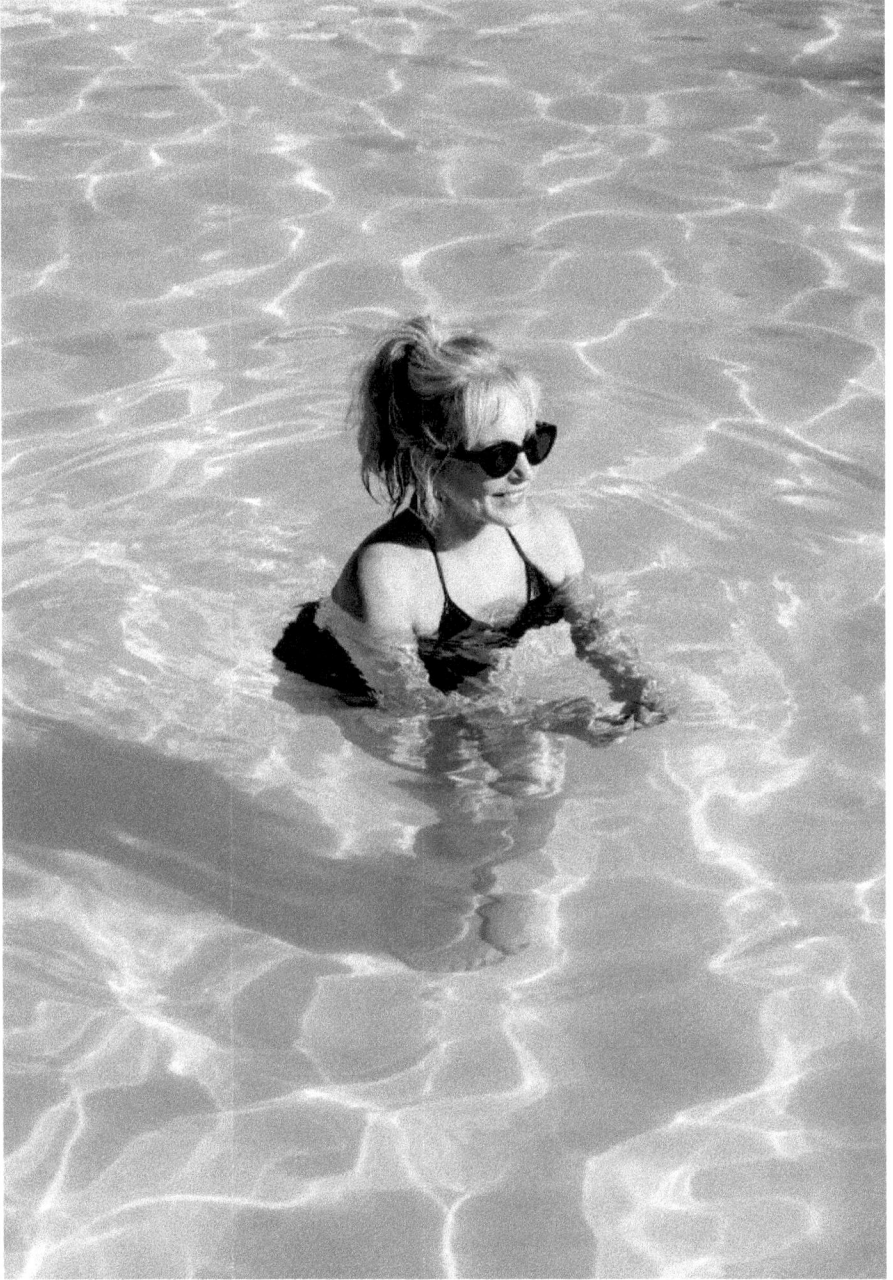

Photo: Lianna Tarantin

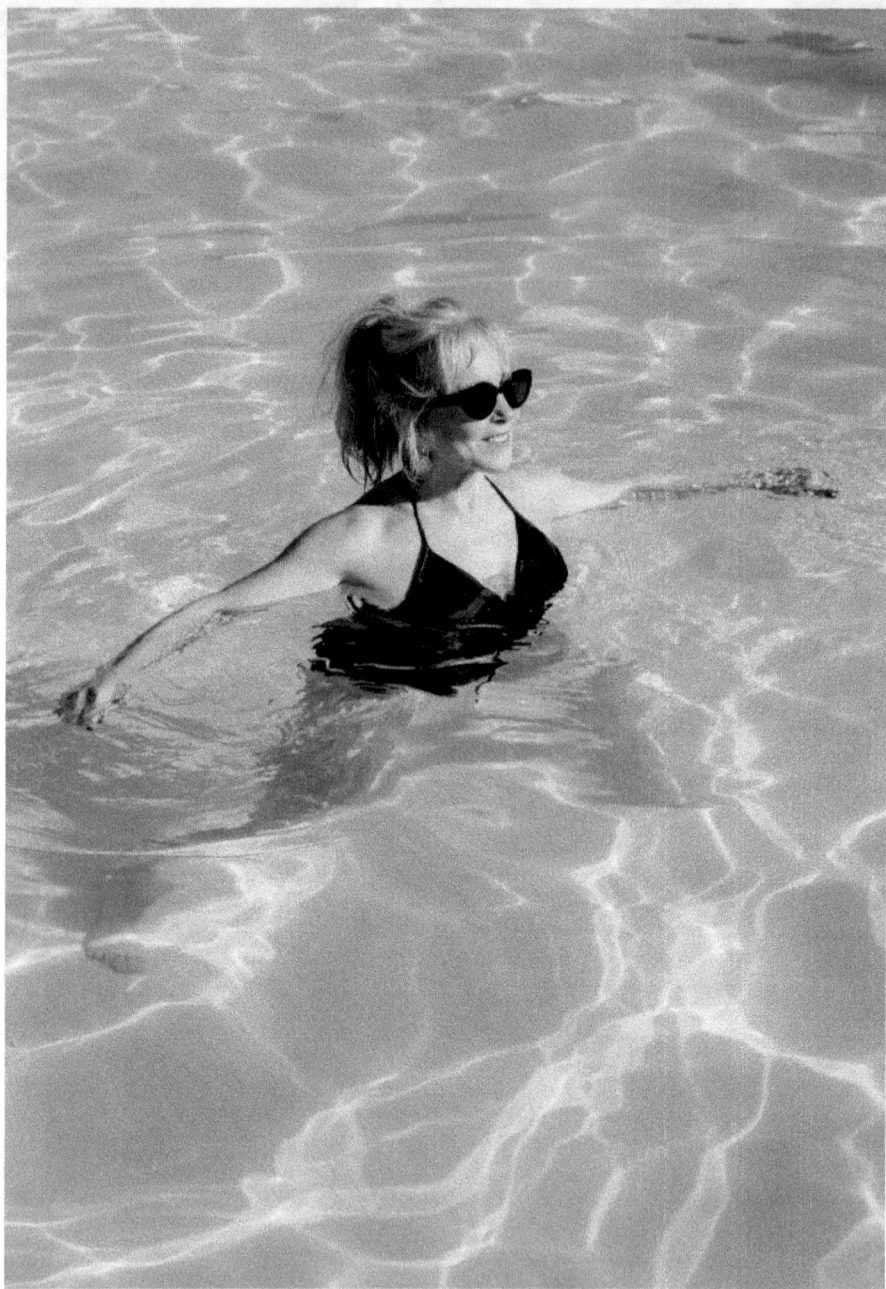

Photo: Lianna Tarantin

2. **Cross-Country Skiing** - Simulate cross-country skiing movements. Slide one foot back while the opposite arm extends forward, then alternate.

3. **Pendulum** - Swing legs side to side with hips squared, maintaining an upright posture. Arm can purposefully move from side to side, or as a triceps exercise.

4. **Rocking Horse** - Alternate kicking one foot forward while the opposite foot kicks back, mimicking a rocking motion. Arms can open wide and contract, like you're giving yourself a big hug.

5. **Kick and Jump** - Perform a forward kick followed by a jump. Alternate legs with each sequence.

6. **Frog Jumps** - Jump upwards from a squat position, bringing heels toward the buttocks, and toward each other, while hips are externally rotated.

7. **Wide Steps** - Take a wide step to one side, bending the knees, then bring the other leg together to meet it.

8. **Soccer Kick** - Kick one leg forward and across the body, leading with the instep of the foot. Alternate legs and challenge yourself, staying vertical or adding a jump.

9. **Skipping with Abandon** - Skip vigorously through the water, lifting knees high and using exaggerated arm movements. This is challenging and so much fun.

Conditioning

1. **Side Leg Lifts** - Stand at the pool's edge; lift one leg to the side and up and then down, maintaining your balance Keep your hips square, toning your thighs.

2. **Side Leg Circles** - Perform circular movements with one leg, keeping the core engaged for stability. To vary for fun, change direction, speed, and lever length.

3. **Hydrants** - While holding onto the pool edge, lift one leg to the side, externally rotating (like a dog at a hydrant, then lower). This is a potent hip "opener."

4. **Donkey Kicks** - From the same position, kick one leg backward, then bring it in and lower it without touching the pool floor.

Cool Down and Stretch

1. **Lower Leg Circles and Ankle Rolls** - Rotate the ankles in slow, deliberate circles to loosen and relax the joints.

2. **Calf Stretch** – Place your hands on a wall about chest level in front of you and feet together. Bring one foot about a step behind your other leg. With the back heel on the floor, bend your front knee, but not more than 90 until you feel a stretch in the back leg. Hold it static, meaning do not bounce, and that the knee in front is not beyond 90 degrees. Hold the stretch for 15 to 30 seconds.

3. **Rib Cage Lunge and Isolation** - Step one foot forward into a lunge while isolating the rib cage, lifting up and moving it side to side.

4. **Shoulder Rolls and Head Tilts** - Roll shoulders gently forward and backward, then tilt the head slowing side to side to stretch the neck. Try to add gentle shoulder roll rhythms: Quick (q) and Slow (s) like: QQS QQS repeat. SSQQS SSQQS rolls back and forward.

5. **Triceps Stretch** - Reach one arm overhead, bend the elbow to touch the opposite shoulder blade, and use the other hand to gently press the elbow for a deeper stretch for 12-15 seconds. Pat yourself on the back for doing a great job.

6. **Hip Circles** – These are good to do when you are warmed up, and for a "stretch interval." Stand grounded with your feet hip-width apart, hands on your hips. Lift up and circle hips slowly to the right around and then circle around left. Variation: Isolate hips diagonal to the front, back to center, back diagonal, center right and left. Luxuriate in the hip release and imagine grounding and lifting up.

7. **Give Yourself A Hug** – For a "peak end," open your heart, bring your arms out to the side, and open wide, stretching your chest, then give yourself a big hug, to celebrate your accomplishments, hold and get a nice back stretch. Water walk with a buddy for a minute and share, "Three Good Things."

8. **Quadriceps Stretch** - Stand on one leg, use the pool wall if you like, bend the knee of the other leg, bringing the heel up towards the buttocks, hold the ankle with your hand, gently pulling the heel closer to the buttocks, keep the knees close together and the back straight. Hold the stretch for 15-30 seconds, then switch legs.

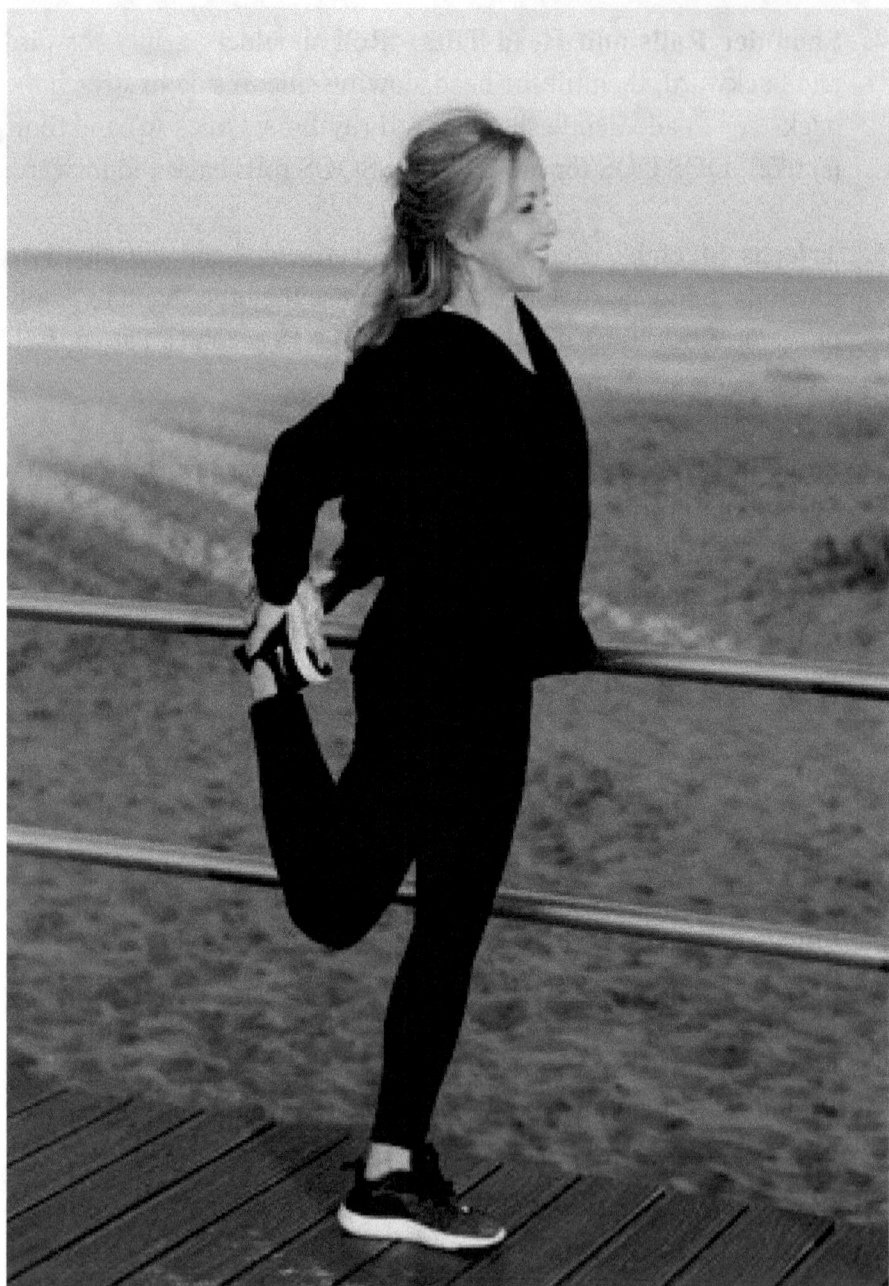

Photo: Lianna Tarantin

Add Variety With These Aqua Fitness Moves

1. **Water Twists** - Stand with feet shoulder-width apart, knees slightly bent. Keep your body in alignment, and on the twist, be sure your knees, ankles, chest, and head are in the same plane. Twist your upper body from side to side, reaching and pulling hands in opposition. Twists help tone the abdominal muscles and improve spinal flexibility. Lower your arms in the water for greater resistance.

2. **Aquatic Boxing** - Perform punching movements underwater, alternating arms. This can include jabs, crosses, uppercuts, and hooks. The water resistance increases the workout intensity for the upper body and core, along with leg and feet stability. Build combinations like: "jab right, cross left, hook right, uppercut left," and move that water like a champion, the champion you are.

3. **High Tail Mule Kicks** – Standing, lift one leg behind you, trying to extend it straight at hip level, then switch legs. Focus on engaging the glutes and hamstrings. This also helps strengthen the lower back and improve balance.

4. **Star Jumps** - Begin in a narrow stance and then jump, extending arms and legs outward into a star shape before returning to the starting position. This plyometric exercise is a dynamic coordination exercise.

5. **Double Leg Lifts** – Advanced. Hold onto the pool edge, float on your back, or stand, and lift both legs together without bending at the knees, then lower them back down to target the lower insertion of the abdominal muscles. Begin by doing one leg at a time to build progression and strength.

6. **Hurdle Jumps** - Simulate powerfully jumping over a hurdle by lifting one knee and the opposite arm as you jump to the side and front. It's a plyometric exercise that's fun when you alternate sides to promote your agility and coordination.

7. **Seahorse Float** - Float vertically with legs together and arms extended down in the water. Use a slow sculling motion with the hands to maintain an upright position. This exercise improves core strength, balance, focus, and relaxation.

8. **Helicopter** - In a standing position, rotate your arms in large circles to create resistance, first in one direction, then the other. This is effective for shoulder mobility and strengthening. For a laugh, perform helicopters in circles.

9. **Pool Planks** - Holding a noodle in front of you with both hands, lean forward, into a plank position with your body straight and toes touching the pool bottom. Hold this position to engage the core. Challenge your strength and balance by adding push up variations. Also try it with your feet off the ground, like a superhero, horizontal with your arms stretched forward, head and neck in alignment. Soar into your strength.

10. **Vertical Knee Raise** - Stand in high waist to chest height water and lift your knees alternately as high as possible, mimicking a marching motion but with emphasis on the height of the knee lift. This move helps strengthen the core and hip flexors. Add arm variations, biceps curls, triceps kickbacks, arm raises.

11. **Aqua Lunges** - Perform forward, side, and backward lunges. The water provides resistance and aids in balance, and safely increases your leg strength.

12. **Zigzag Jog** – Jog, lead, dance, run, and play in a zigzag pattern across the pool, changing directions quickly to improve agility and cardiovascular fitness.

13. **Penguin Waddle** - With feet close together, take small side steps. Keep your body straight and move quickly to create a waddling effect, which helps with hip flexibility and lateral movement.

Stretching *Splash*Dance

In *Splash*Dance, like in life, stretching is an integral component of our fitness. The importance of flexibility cannot be underscored, along with mobility for overall health and performance. Incorporating stretches after the initial thermal warm-up allows you to work with tissues that respond more effectively when warm, rather than cold. Think of your muscles like taffy. If you pull, or stretch taffy when it's cold, it's hard; when you warm the taffy, there is greater ease and malleability. Warmth enhances the effectiveness of your stretches, reducing the risk of injury and improving your flexibility. Furthermore, integrating flexibility training as intervals during workouts ensures that muscles remain limber and responsive throughout the session, maximizing the benefits of each movement. Concluding your *Splash*Dance with a final luxuriating stretch helps to cool down your body, supports muscle recovery, and increases relaxation.

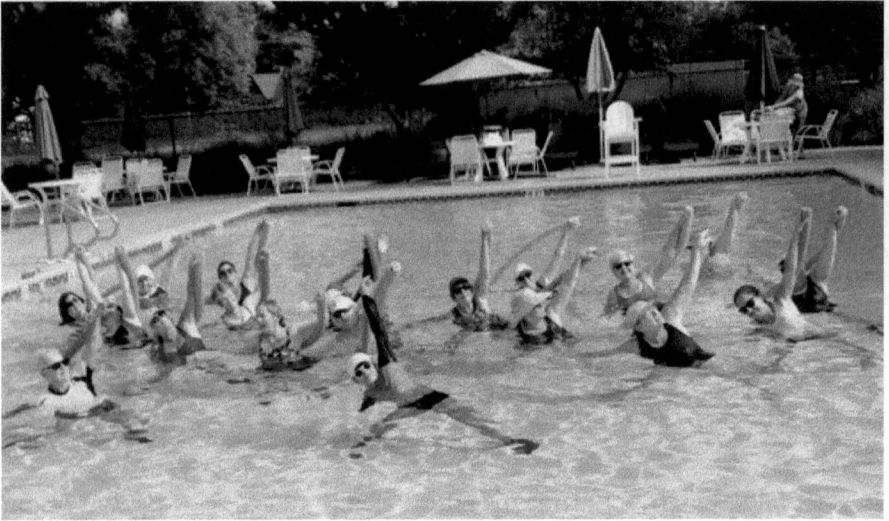

Photo at Fairway Mews, Spring Lake Heights, NJ

Stretching Techniques in the Pool

1. **Standing Stretches**: Perform arm sweeps, side bends, and leg stretches while standing in high-waist or shoulder-deep water to utilize the water's resistance and buoyancy, enhance the stretch, and support the body.

2. **Sitting Stretches on a Step or Ledge**: Sit on a submerged step or ledge to perform lower back stretches, hamstring stretches, and ankle circles. This allows you to target stretching muscles with gentle support from the water.

3. **Poolside Stretches**: Use the pool's edge for support while performing calf stretches, standing quadriceps stretches, or leaning forward for deeper stretches in the hips and lower back.

4. **Floating Stretches**: For a deeply relaxing stretch, use pool noodles or flotation devices to support your body in a floating position, allowing for unrestricted movement and a unique stretching experience that only water can provide.

By incorporating these stretching methods, and the "Cool Down and Stretch" exercises in the previous chapter into *Splash*Dance, you'll enjoy a comprehensive benefit and approach to flexibility that complements the cardiovascular and strength components of the program. This training leads to improved range of motion, decreased muscle stiffness, and enhanced fluidity in your daily movements. Practice stretching to boost your mind-body wisdom, and to feel fit and fabulous.

Aerobics: *The Key to Fitness*

Engage in aerobic exercises with *Splash*Dance and witness a transformation in your physical and mental health. Aerobics means "with oxygen," and consists of the continuous rhythmic movement of major muscle groups. Other aerobic activities include brisk walking, running, bicycling, swimming, and dance. Aerobics are pivotal in strengthening your cardiovascular system, enhancing brain health, and improving overall vitality.

Benefits of Aerobics Training

1. **Improves Cardiovascular Health**: Lowers the risk of heart disease by improving heart health through regular aerobic activity.

2. **Blood Pressure Reduction**: Regular aerobic exercise helps in lowering blood pressure, contributing to cardiovascular health.

3. **Stress Alleviation**: Effectively reduces tension, fatigue, and stress, enhancing mental well-being.

4. **Osteoporosis Prevention**: Maintains and potentially increases bone mass, reducing the risk of osteoporosis.

5. **Improved Body Composition**: Promotes a healthier body composition by increasing muscle mass and decreasing body fat.

6. **Enhanced Oxygen Utilization**: Increases VO2 max, which is the maximum amount of oxygen the body can utilize during intense exercise.

7. **Boosted Self-Concept**: Engaging in regular aerobic exercise can significantly improve self-esteem and overall self-image.

8. **Increased Energy Stores**: Boosts muscle glycogen stores, which are critical for sustained physical activity and energy.

9. **Improved Cardiac Efficiency**: Enhances heart function by increasing stroke volume and reducing resting heart rate, leading to more efficient heart performance.

10. **Enhanced Respiratory Capacity**: Improves the overall capacity and efficiency of the breathing process.

11. **Improved Lipid Profile**: Brings about positive changes in blood lipid levels, decreasing fats that can lead to heart disease.

12. **Elevated Athletic Performance**: Enhances endurance, strength, and overall athletic performance, making everyday activities easier and less taxing.

13. Aerobic training enhances brain health: By promoting neuroplasticity and neurogenesis, processes that enable the brain to create new neural connections and generate new brain cells, improving cognitive function and memory. Aerobics also increases the production of Brain-Derived Neurotrophic Factor (BDNF), a protein that supports neuron growth and survival, crucial for learning and mental health. Aerobic training also improves executive function, which includes cognitive processes such as planning, attention, problem-solving, and multitasking, along with better decision-making, increased focus, and improved mental flexibility.

Each of these points illustrates how aerobic training, especially within the dynamic and engaging environment of *Splash*Dance, not only serves physical health but also enriches mental and emotional well-being, making it a cornerstone of a holistic approach to fitness.

The American Council on Sports Medicine recommends training aerobically 3-5 times weekly for at least 30 minutes or more (or a minimum of three 10-minute sessions, can significantly boost your health within just a few weeks. So, catch the wave, keep moving, and watch your whole well-being improve pretty quickly.

Aerobic exercises use the large muscle groups of your body (arms and legs) while moving then continuously and rhythmically starting with 10 -20 minutes to start and build up progression. Aerobic activities, like *Splash*Dance include swimming, dancing, brisk walking, jogging, sports like cycling, soccer, basketball, and cross-country skiing.

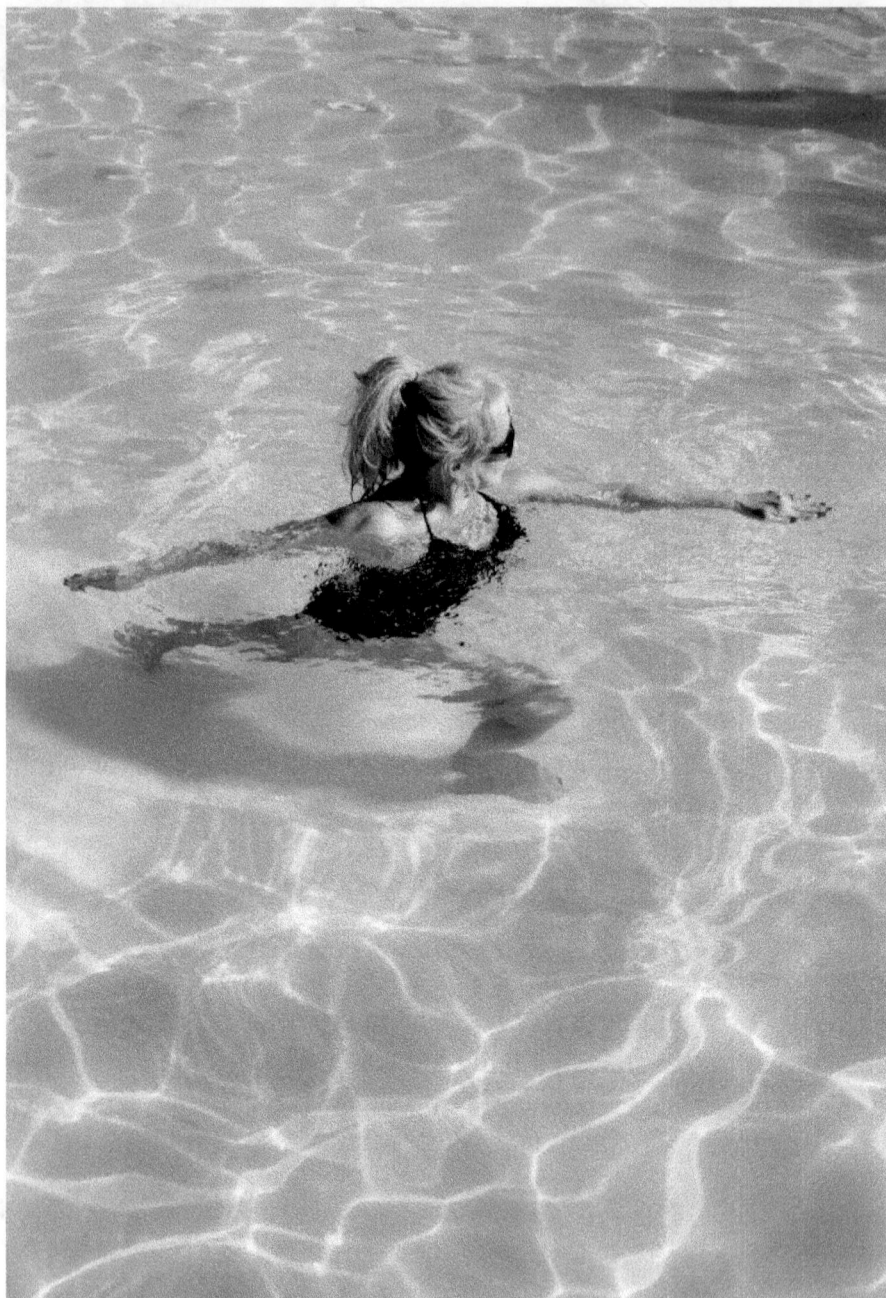

Photo: Lianna Tarantin

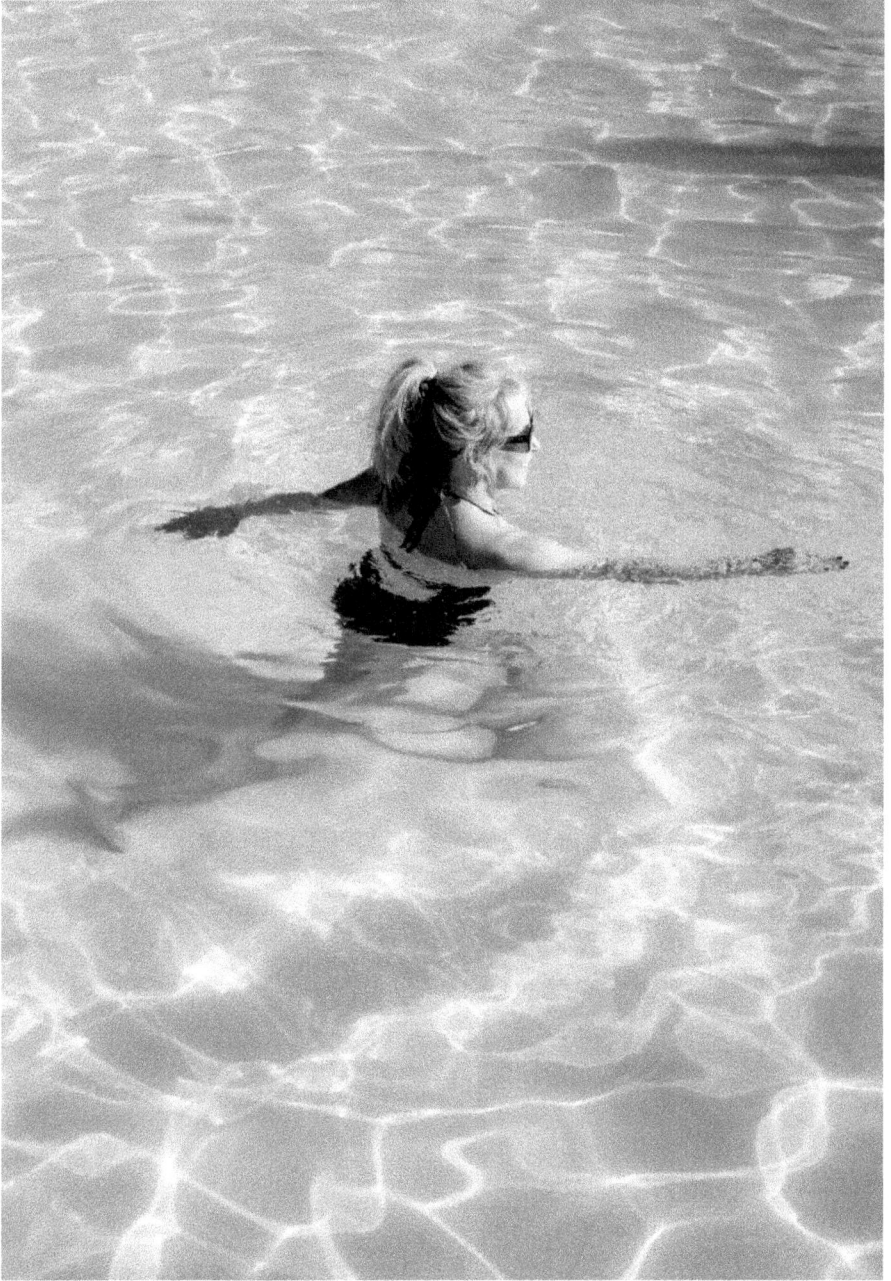

Photo: Lianna Tarantin

Ski the Waters: Unleash Your Cross-Country Pool Potential: A favorite in aqua fitness, Cross Country Skiing offers a comprehensive cardiovascular workout that simulates the movements of snow skiing. Here's how you can perform it in the pool in either shallow (waist to chest height) or deep-water:

1. **Starting Position:** Stand in chest-deep water with your feet hip-width apart. Engage your core to maintain an upright posture. In deep water, it's recommended to use a floatation device to help you really engage in the moves.

2. **The Movement:** Slide one foot backward while the opposite arm reaches forward. Then switch, sliding the opposite foot back as the corresponding arm comes forward.

3. **Arm Action:** Use a coordinated arm swing, pushing water with each stroke to increase resistance and maximize the workout.

4. **Focus on Form:** Keep your movements smooth and rhythmic, ensuring each leg and arm extends fully to benefit from each motion's stretch and strength aspects.

Benefits:

- Provides a full-body workout, engaging legs, arms, and core.

- Enhances cardiovascular health through sustained, rhythmic activity.

- Offers low-impact (shallow water) and non-impact (deep-water) resistance, ideal for joint health and is suitable for all fitness levels.

- It's fun, challenging and feels great!

Additional Moves for To Boost Your Energy and Power

1. **LeapFrog** - Jump up from a squat position, lifting your knees high towards the chest, then land softly back into a squat. This move increases heart rate and strengthens the lower body.

2. **Aqua Stride Jump** – Add a small jump while performing the stride movements, with each switch of the legs to increase intensity and a plyometric element.

3. **Slalom Jumps** - Jump side to side with feet together, hip-width apart, keeping your knees slightly bent. Simulating downhill skiing, it's excellent for lateral movement, agility, and energy boost.

4. **Aquatic Tuck Jumps** - Jump up, bringing knees up toward your chest, then extend legs back down before landing. This high-intensity move is great for your core strength, vitality, and has perfect plyometric powerhouse potential.

5. **The Cheerleader** - Perform three small jumps with a clap under the knee at the top of each jump, followed by a high jump on the fourth count, lifting the knees as high as possible. This fun, high-energy move boosts your heart rate and your spirit.

6. **Sweeper** - Extend one leg out to the front and then sweep it side to side across the water. This works core and inner/outer thigh muscles along with balance.

Integrate some of these additional moves into your aqua fitness sessions to provide you with variety, challenge, and a full range of benefits.

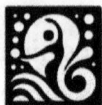

Questions for Reflection and Positive Action

1. **Technique Evaluation**: After practicing some of the moves described, like the Leaps or Frog Jumps, which exercises did you enjoy and which were most challenging? How might mastering these moves help you feel?

2. **Community Sharing**: Have fun practicing one move from each phase (thermal warmup, aerobics, conditioning, cooldown, stretching) with an aqua fitness friend or classmate. What are your favorite moves?.

3. **Benefits of Aerobic Training**: How can engaging in regular aerobic exercise, such as *Splash*Dance, improve your cardiovascular health and vitality?

4. **Mental Health and Aerobics**: Discuss how aerobic activities, including *Splash*Dance, enhance brain health, specifically focusing on the roles of neuroplasticity, neurogenesis, and Brain-Derived Neurotrophic Factor (BDNF).

5. **Progress Tracking**: Set an aqua fitness goal. What specific steps will you take to achieve this goal, and how will you measure your progress over time?

CHAPTER 18

Aqua Rhythms, Fun Formations, and Group Dynamics

Sometimes in the waves of change we find our true direction.

- Unknown

Participating in *Splash*Dance as a group fitness activity transcends conventional physical training; it cultivates a holistic environment where physical, social, emotional, and psychological well-being synergistically thrive. Engaging in rhythmic group exercises where "together you are moving as one," immerses you in a phenomenon known as "communitas"—a profound spirit of community, solidarity, and connection. This is where moving as a group, we become "bigger" than ourselves as an individual. Aqua Formations' synchronized movements not only elevate individual fitness but also amplify collective well-being, transforming each session into a vibrant journey of vitality and joy shared among all participants. This chapter explores how these dynamic formations foster an exhilarating sense of unity and exhilaration, making every *Splash*Dance experience a celebration of communal health and happiness.

Optimizing Aquatic Spaces for Dynamic *Splash*Dance Formations

Each pool offers a unique opportunity to design effective, energizing, and engaging formations based on its specific layout. You can assess the pool's design and ways to navigate, including from shallow to deep water, using lanes to create traveling patterns, or in creating formations to continuously challenge your abilities. Engaging in inventive patterns and formations are fun ways to optimize your resistance. These increase drag forces, along with adding a dose of camaraderie and some laughs.

Aqua Power Formations: A Symphony of Turbulence in the Water

Aqua Power formations bring a new dimension to aqua fitness, blending the laws of physics with the sheer joy of dance, exercise, and sport. These formations leverage the unique properties of water—buoyancy, pressure, and resistance—to create a multilevel exercise experience that's as beneficial as it is delightful. Here's a guide to some of the most dynamic and engaging formations:

- **Jellyfish**: Move towards and away from the center in a fluid, undulating motion, mimicking the natural movement of a jellyfish.

- **Pinwheel**: This formation involves directional changes and both forward and backward movements, and spins, adding a layer of complexity and fun.

- **Conga Line**: Following the leader single file, or 2 x 2, this incorporates runs, skips, hops, and a conga line formation, "1, 2, 3, kick, 1, 2, 3 kick" weaving through the water.

- **Juicy Jitterbug**: Encourage partners or groups to mirror each other's movements, adding spins, varying movements, all while staying attuned to the rhythms.

- **Slalom Run**: Simulate a skiing experience across the pool with a gentler landing, by jumping from side to side, to encourage strength and knee flexibility.

Expanded Formation Choices

Add these creative and social elements for a rich, exhilarating vitality-promoting experience. To maintain freshness and challenge, here is an extended list of formations that can be incorporated into your repertoire:

- **Circle the Wagons**: Circle up and create waves. It's challenging to maintain your position against the water's movement.

- **Swing Your Partner**: Incorporate square dancing elements, fostering interaction, coordination, fellowship, and fun.

- **Stroll Down the Lane: Dick Clark American Bandstand Style:** Form two   parallel lines, facing each other. At the top of the line, participant pairs move down the center lane with their partner, reminiscent of the classic American Bandstand. Two at a time, glide down the lane to the end, performing your favorite moves together before returning to your outer lines. Keep your core engaged to contribute to the smoothness of your glide. Personalize your stroll by adding moves and elements that match your style and the music. You can stride, ski, twirl, dip, or groove to the beat before continuing your stroll.

- **Grand Right and Left**: Introduces elements of traditional square dance that are challenging, structured, and fun. Here's how to do this formation: Start in a square, facing your partner. Extend your right hand to the opposite dancer, switch to the left hand for the next, and continue alternating hands. Move around the square, passing each dancer, until you return to your original position with your partner. The sequence ends when you meet your partner again.

Cool Down and Relaxation Techniques

Conclude your session with a dedicated relaxation and cool-down phase:

Toes in Walking: Walk with a pigeon-toed gait to stretch your calves.

Esther Williams: Perform flowing movements to activate the core and calm your body. With aqua barbells or a noodle supporting you, bring your knees to your chest and move your extended legs to one side, and repeat to the other side.

Sunshine Super Stretch for Abdominals and Back: Begin floating on your back with your body fully extended, arms at your sides. From floating, perform a tuck by drawing your knees towards your chest, wrapping your arms around knees briefly, squeezing your abdominal muscles tightly. Quickly extend your arms and legs outwards, stretching them as far as possible. You can also keep your limbs close to the water's surface, engaging your core to maintain balance and stability. As you alternate between the tuck and the extended stretch, focus on engaging your core muscles throughout. This will help strengthen your abdominal area. Continue in a smooth, controlled manner, and try to keep the transitions between the tuck and stretch as fluid as possible, maintaining a consistent rhythm.

Massage Circle: Gently give and receive an encouraging shoulder or neck rub.

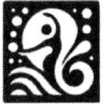

Questions for Reflection and Positive Action

1. **Community Experience Reflection**: How might participating in group formations like the "Pinwheel" or "Conga Line" enhance your sense of community and connectedness?

2. **Formation Exploration**: Can you create a new formation or modify an existing one? Think about how your formation could foster greater interaction and fun among people.

3. **Personal and Social -being Integration**: After trying dynamic formations, reflect on momemts that may lift your spirits, and make you feel like you are part of something "larger than yourself.

CHAPTER 19

Strengthen and Tone - Arms and Upper Body Aqua Choreography

Water does not resist. Water flows. When you plunge your hand into it, all you feel is a caress."

- Margaret Atwood, Essayist, Environmental Activist.

Aqua upper body exercises and strength training in the water offer a unique environment as the water provides resistance to challenge your muscles while reducing impact on your joints. Here are some aqua upper body strength exercises:

1. **Water Push-Ups**: Stand facing the pool wall, your arms extended forward and your hands resting on the pool deck. Lower your body by bending your elbows and leaning towards the wall. Push yourself back up and target your chest, triceps, and shoulders, Lower your heels, bringing the toes up (dorsiflexion) to powerfully stretch your calves.

2. **Water Arm Circles**: Stand in shoulder-deep water with your feet shoulder-width apart. Extend your arms out to the sides at shoulder level. Begin making small circles with your arms, gradually increasing the size of the circles. Reverse the direction after a set amount of time. Arm circles engage the shoulders and improve shoulder mobility. The deeper the arms, the greater the resistance.

3. **Water Triceps Dips**: Sit on the edge of the pool with your hands gripping the pool deck on either side of your hips. Slide your bot-

tom off the edge and lower your body by bending your elbows. Keep your back close to the pool wall and your legs extended in front of you. Push yourself back up to the starting position.

4. **Water Bicep Curls**: Stand in chest-deep water with your feet hip-width apart. Hold water dumbbells in each hand with your palms facing forward. Keeping your elbows close to your body, curl your hands towards your shoulders and then lower them back down. Bicep curls target the biceps and forearms

5. **Water Chest Press**: Stand with feet shoulder-width apart in chest or waist-height water. Place your hands (aqua dumbells or other buoyant object), at chest or shoulder level, with your palms facing forward. Extend your arms straight ahead, pushing the water, and then return to starting position. These mighty presses engage your deltoids, triceps, and upper back muscles. Vary by alternating arms, pressing to the side or down or alternating speed and force.

6. **Water Lateral Raises**: Stand with your feet shoulder-width apart in chest-deep water. Hold water dumbells by your sides with your palms facing inward. Raise your arms out to the sides until they are parallel to the water, then lower them back down. Lateral raises primarily target the deltoid muscles.

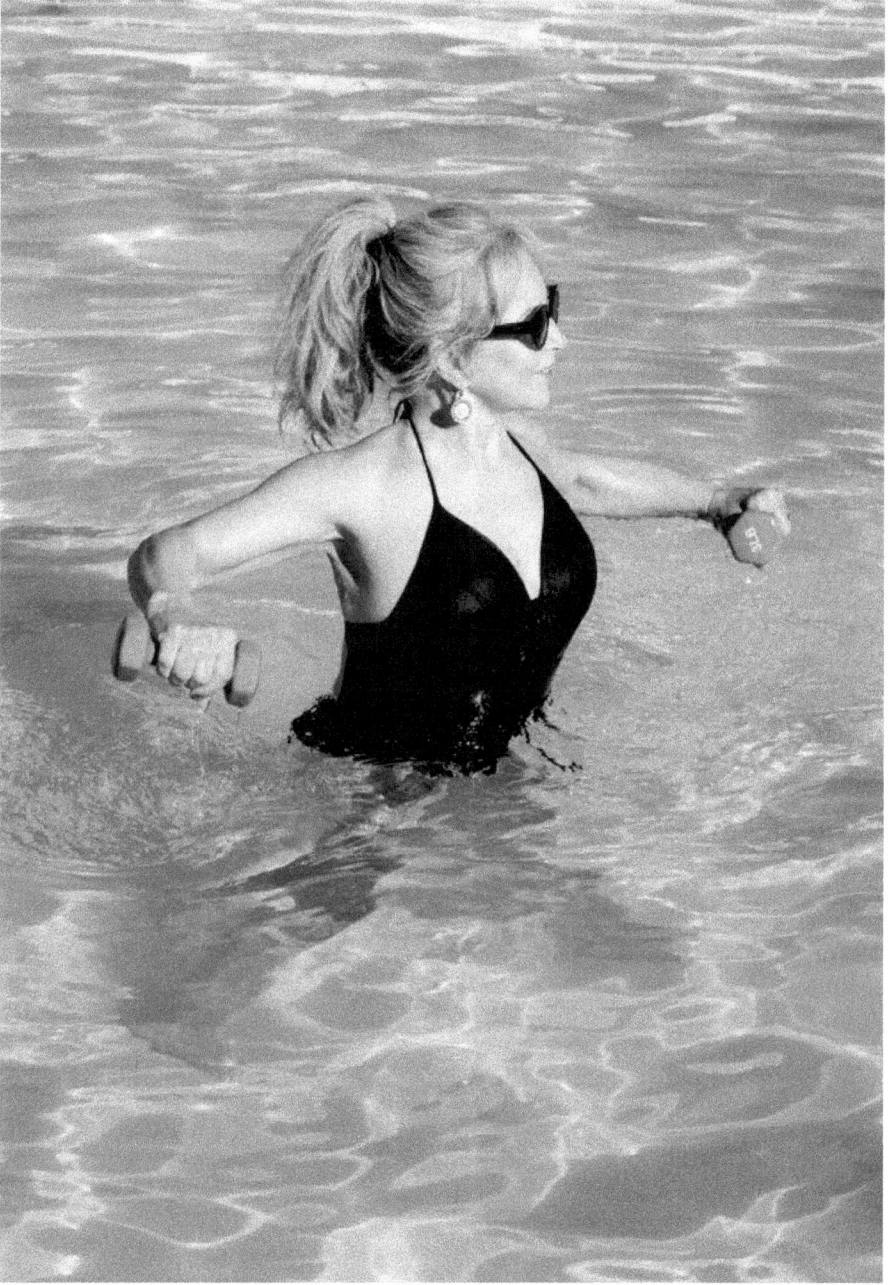

Photo: Lianna Tarantin

7. **Water Punches**: Stand with your feet hip-width apart and slightly bend your knees. Extend your arms out in front of you, keeping them submerged in the water. Alternate punching forward with each arm, focusing on speed and power. This exercise works the shoulders, chest, and arms.

8. **Water Upright Rows:** Upright rows in the pool are an effective strength-building exercise that involves standing in shoulder-depth water and performing a rowing motion by pulling your hands upwards towards your chest, elbows out. This exercise targets the shoulders, back, and arms, leveraging the water's resistance to enhance muscle tone and strength. The buoyancy of the water reduces joint stress, making it ideal for participants of all fitness levels in the *Splash*Dance program.

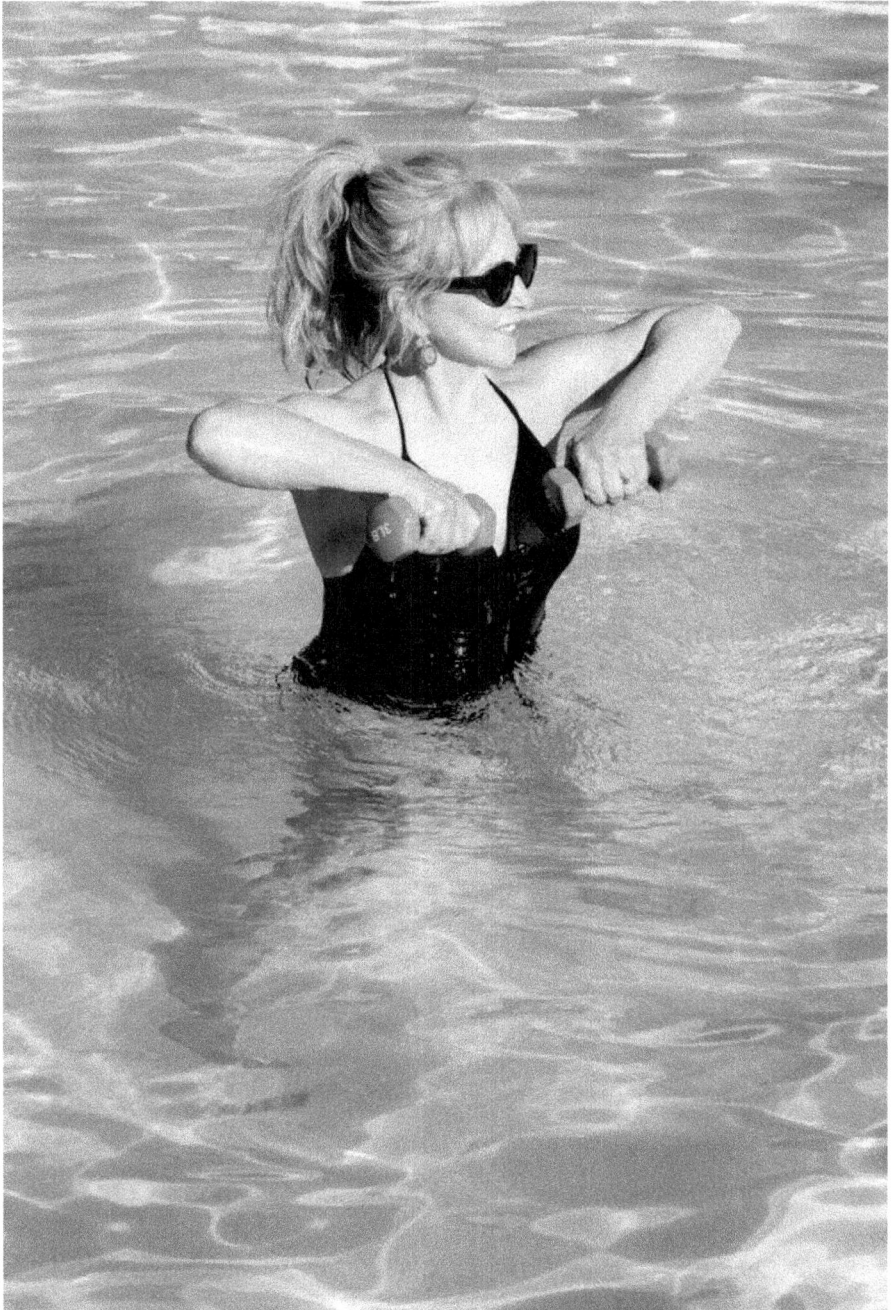

Photo: Lianna Tarantin

Integrating various arm positions and choreographed movements into *Splash*Dance not only injects freshness and variety but also enhances the effectiveness of your upper body workouts. You can keep things engaging and challenging by varying the complexity and intensity of your movements. Arms play a crucial role by either assisting or resisting the momentum of the lower body and allow for adjustments in your training intensity. Additionally, arm movements help stabilize the body and maintain proper alignment. For instance, while a backward jump is facilitated by cupping the hands and pulling the arms forward, incorporating breaststroke movements significantly intensifies the exercise. Exploring diverse arm techniques in the pool increases complexity and also adds a fun element as you discover new ways to move and groove in the water.

Webs: The term "webs" can refer to the natural spread of the fingers that mimics the function of webbed aqua fitness gloves. When you spread your fingers wide during exercises, the surface area of your hands increases, which adds resistance as you move through the water. This technique helps strengthen the muscles of your arms and upper body by maximizing the water's resistance. Using the hands as "webs" is a simple yet effective method to enhance the intensity without the need for additional equipment. This approach leverages the properties of water for resistance training, helping to improve muscle tone, endurance, and overall fitness.

Table 1: Customizing Your Training Intensity

This table provides a clear guide on adjusting the intensity of exercises in *Splash*Dance by manipulating surface area, force speed, size of movement, and travel pace.

Intensity	Surface Area	Force Speed	Size of Move	Travel
Low	Slicing webs	Push lightly, softly	Small moves, keep arms & legs flexed	Go easy, slow
Moderate	Cupping webs	Push harder, faster	Reach farther, increasing range of motion without locking joints	Pick up tempo, push harder
High	Webs open	Push with power & force	Full range of motion, arms & legs extended	Push with maximum force and speed

At a Glance Arm Choreography

This is a chart of "Aqua Arm Moves" along with descriptions. Try each of these for 45 seconds while standing, walking, or water running:

Aqua Arm Move	Description
Crawl	Perform a freestyle swimming arm motion, alternating arms in a forward circular motion enhancing shoulder mobility and upper body strength.
Fin Arms (Straight)	Extend arms straight out to the sides and slice through the water like fins, providing resistance training for the shoulders and upper back.
Figure 8	Move arms in a continuous figure-eight pattern underwater, improving coordination and engaging both the core and upper body muscles. This is also called "sculling," from water ballet.
Open and Close Arms - Expand and Contract	Start with arms extended wide, then bring them together in front of you (give yourself a hug) and back out, utilizing the water's resistance to strengthen your chest and back.
Twist, with Hands at the Side	Keep your arms straight and close to the body, and twist your torso from side to side, engaging the core and obliques.
Push Arms Straight Down and Up (Upright Row)	Push arms straight down through the water, then lift them up in an upright rowing motion, training the shoulders, upper back, and biceps.
Breaststroke	Perform the arm motion, pushing water from the chest, outwards and then sweeping inwards, ideal for chest, shoulders, and upper back conditioning.
Roll Arms and Shoulders	Rotate the arms and shoulders in circular movements to loosen and strengthen your shoulder joints, enhancing flexibility and reducing tension.

Visualize and apply the different arm movements.

Remember to warm up before starting these exercises. Adjust your intensity based on your fitness level, and your desired outcome. Gradually increase the repetitions or resistance as you get stronger. It's very important to maintain good form and control.

These are many arm exercises that work well with power leg moves such as cross-country skiing, jumping jacks, jogging, and lunges. Here are some more for you to try:

Aqua Arm Move	Description
Triceps Press To The Side	Performed with a jog or jumping jack, begin with your elbows lifted to the sides. Extend your forearms out to the side, turning the palms to face upward, tightening the triceps during the extension. Flex the elbow, bringing the forearms in front of the body, again turning the palms upward.
Lateral Press	Begin with arms lifted shoulder height in front of the body. Pull the arms out to the sides with the elbows just slightly bent, palms facing to the back. Return to the starting position, turning the palms to face together. Great with lunges.
Shoulder Extension /Hyperextension	Begin with the arms shoulder height in front of the body. With the elbows slightly bent and palms facing down, pull the arms down to the sides or behind the body. Palms turn face up as you return.
Punch and Pull	Begin with the arms lifted in front of the body below shoulder height, elbows slightly bent. Pull the elbows back behind the body, squeezing the shoulder blades tightly together. Punch the arms forward, moving both arms together and alternating arms across your body.

As your technique, form and endurance improves, you will be able to use power moves to maintain training heart rate throughout the aerobics segment, using a few jogs or other such movements simply as transitions. As you feel more confident, you can incorporate combinations that are fun, add variety and develop your coordination as well. Play and be creative; just don't compromise safety.

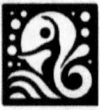

Questions for Reflection and Positive Action

1. **Arm Choreography Variations**: Reflect on the different arm movements described, such as Crawl, Fin Arms, and Figure 8. Which of these arm choreographies do you find most fun or challenging, and how do they contribute to your upper body toning and strength?

2. **Effectiveness of Upper Body Exercises**: Considering exercises like Water Push-Ups and Water Dips, how effective do you find these in targeting and strengthening your upper body muscles?

3. **Muscle Engagement**: Do you notice any differences in muscle engagement when performing standing versus buoyant abdominal exercises in the water?

CHAPTER 20

Duality - Exploring Opposition and Muscular Balance in *Splash*Dance

This concept of opposition is particularly effective in aqua fitness, where the resistance of the water amplifies the benefits by adding a natural challenge to the oppositional movements; this enhances the training's intensity and effectiveness. In dance and aqua fitness training, "opposition" refers to the concept of moving different parts of the body in contrasting directions to create balance and harmony. This principle is commonly used to enhance stability, coordination, and the efficiency of movements. For example, when one arm moves forward, the opposite leg extends backward, helping to maintain balance and ensuring a full-body workout. Cross-country skiing is a perfect example.

The benefits of using opposition in dance and aqua fitness include:

1. **Improved Balance:** By engaging opposing muscles and limbs, you develop better control over your body, and enhance your ability to balance and perform movements.

2. **Enhanced Coordination:** Practicing movements that incorporate opposition help to coordinate limbs and torso movements more effectively, leading to smoother and more integrated actions.

3. **Increased Muscle Engagement:** Oppositional movements ensure that various muscle groups are activated, leading to a more comprehensive workout that can improve overall muscle tone and strength.

4. **Reduced Risk of Injury:** By promoting balanced muscle activation and improving overall body awareness, opposition helps to distribute the physical stress of movement more evenly, reducing the likelihood of overuse injuries.

5. **Greater Efficiency:** Opposition can make movements more energy-efficient, as it leverages the body's natural dynamics, helping practitioners perform better with less fatigue.

Experiment with different arm/leg combinations. One rule to remember: If you lift a leg behind the body, the same arm or both arms should come forward to prevent stress on the lower back.

Opposition and Muscular Balance

Strength training is one of the best things you can do to protect your lifetime fitness. The water provides resistance in all directions, so we can focus and vary the force of the movement. The goal here is in designing an exercise program to provide muscle balance within each workout. Movement in opposite directions, traveling forward, backward, and laterally through the water, and changing your walking or striding frequently, is an excellent strategy for success.

Varying your arm and leg patterns adds creativity and provides a more effective whole-body workout as well. Arms can assist or resist the lower body's momentum and thereby change intensity level, but they can also be used to stabilize the body and maintain correct alignment.

Muscular Balance and Muscular Imbalance

Muscle groups often work in pairs in order to first flex and then extend a part of the body at a joint. A good example of the flexor/extensor pairs are the hamstring/quadriceps muscle groups. The hamstrings (back of the thigh) bend the knee, and the quadriceps (front of thigh) straighten (extend) this joint. Muscle balance is achieved when both muscle groups in a pair are developed to the same degree. Imbalance, resulting from over-development or underdevelopment of one member of the pair, can cause poor posture, pain, tendon tightness and eventual misalignment of the body's framework. Another bonus of aqua fitness upper body training, is that when we activate the muscles in the water, as in biceps curls, we simultaneously train the triceps due to the water's properties (action/reaction).

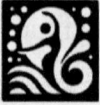

Questions for Reflection and Positive Action

1. **Personal Application**: Can you try to practice and reflect on the principle of opposition? Notice any potential improvements on your balance, energy, and attention.

2. **Creative Experimentation**: Have fun trying to create and practice a new set of movements applying the principle of opposition, like extending your left arm forward while your right leg moves backward, then switching. How does varying these movements affect your intensity, muscle engagement, and coordination?

3. **Muscle Awareness**: Considering the concept of muscle balance, identify any signs of muscular imbalance you might be experiencing. What could you integrate into your routine to address these imbalances?

CHAPTER 21

Priming Athletic Performance and Adding Powerful Plyometrics

For high-performance athletes, fitness athletes, fitness advocates and enthusiasts, *Splash*Dance offers high-level cross-training, embracing variations like manipulating short and long levers, speed, and resistance for you to train "full out." *SplashDance* is the perfect cross-training complement. It also offers the chance to execute plyometrics, without the risk of an overuse injury. Athletes, and beginners alike, can get a power-packed workout in the pool by understanding and utilizing the physics of the water's properties by adding plyometrics' explosive movements. Listen to your amazing body, heart and mind. Play and experiement to challenge yourself and to meet your athletic goals.

Athletic Ability - Coaching Athletes for the National Aerobics Championship: As a U.S. Head Judge, and then coach and trainer for the National Aerobics Championship (NAC) in its heyday, I would bring my talented, high-performance athletes to the pool to cross train, adding dynamic aqua fitness training to the mix. The novelty of a water environment provided both power and protection for improving these athlete's endurance, flexibility, muscular strength, dynamic power, and relaxation.

My NAC champion, Masters Individual Women's multi-medalist, Karen Lenhart Cook, and I were speaking about our time coaching and training together in the pool. Karen, an amazing athlete, professional fitness instructor, dental hygienist, and wonderful human, shared "Training in the pool was great cross training, forgiving on the joints, but excellent resistance work from the water. It kept up my level of fitness and movement while allowing healing so I could come back stronger. I remember running and doing plyometrics like jump splits and straddles to boost my power and flexibility. The water also calmed me down and gave me confidence to train at a very high level."

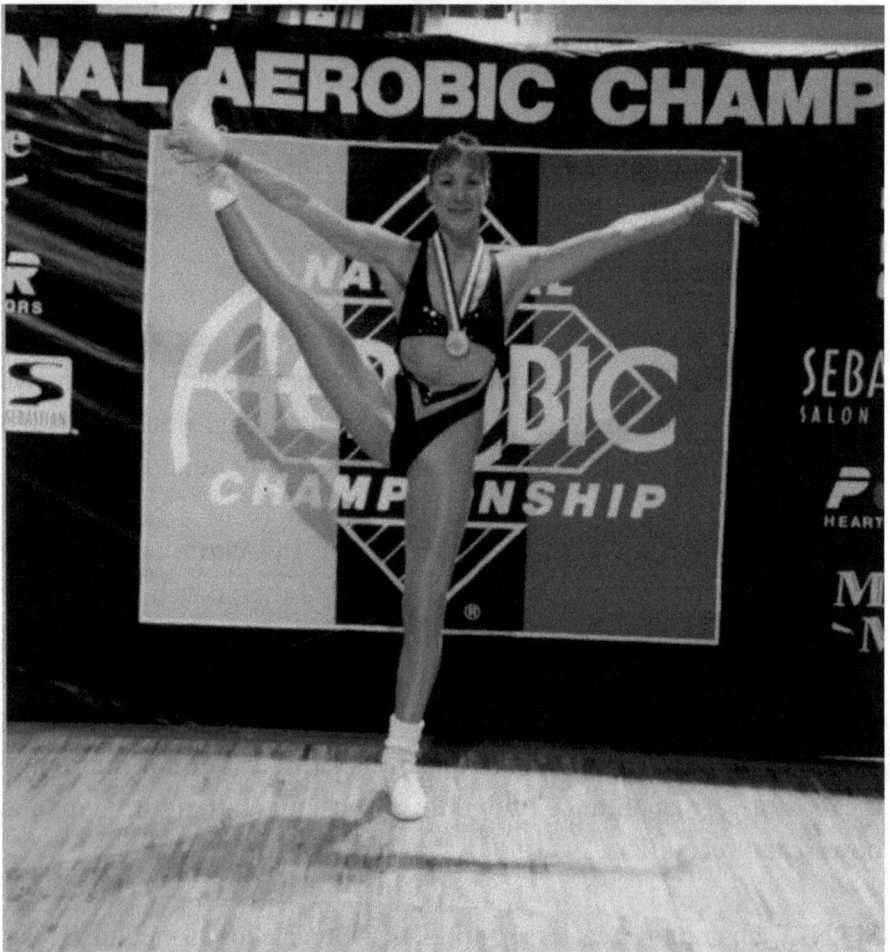

Karen Lenhart Cook, National Aerobic Champion Women's Master's Medalist, 1996

The pool was a great place to train these highest-level competitive athletes. Aqua fitness enhanced the athlete's performance, boosted their muscular strength, muscular endurance, and anaerobic power while boosting range of motion, agility, and balance. The pool was a safe place to practice precarious lifts, imagine, play, and perform competition choreography full-out. There was great joy among the athletes moving freely in the water at a very high level. I think champion Karen Lenhart Cook said it best, "The water is powerful, incredibly therapeutic and elicits happy feelings with lots of smiles and laughter."

The Explosive Power of Pool Plyometrics:

Plyometrics, also known as "jump training," is where the body exerts maximum force in short intervals of time. The goal is in increasing power, and to focus on learning to move a muscle extension to a contraction in an explosive manner such as specialized varied jumping moves like these:

1. **Airjack**: Start with feet together and arms at your sides. Jump up, using the water's resistance, spread your legs and arms out to the sides like a traditional jumping jack, then bring them back to starting position as you land in the water.

2. **Tucks**: Begin in a standing position in the water. Jump up while pulling your knees up to your chest. Use your hands to draw the knees in closer for added intensity, then extend back to standing as you land.

3. **Frogs**: From a standing position in deeper water, explode upwards, pulling your knees outward and upward towards your elbows, with

the soles of the feet toward each other, before returning to standing upon landing.

4. **Pikes**: Advanced. Jump up from a standing position, extending your legs forward while trying to keep them straight and parallel to the pool bottom. Reach your arms towards your toes, then return to standing.

5. **Straddles**: Jump up from a standing position, split your legs to the sides while airborne as wide as possible (like doing a side split in mid-air), and reach your arms towards your toes, then close the legs and return to standing upon landing.

6. **Leaps**: From a standing position, perform a forceful forward jump, driving one knee up while extending the other leg back, much like a dancer's leap, then switch legs and repeat.

7. **Split Leaps**: Leap forward from a standing position, extending the front leg forward and the back leg backward into a split position while airborne, then land back into a staggered stance.

8. **Pirouettes**: Stand on one leg, using the buoyancy to help lift the other leg slightly, then spin around on the supporting foot, using your arms to help control and stabilize the movement.

9. **Cheerleader Jumps**: Begin in chest-high water with feet shoulder-width apart. Stand, then explosively jump up, placing your arms into a "V" shape at your side and lifting your knees towards the chest. Aim for a "V" shape with your body at the jump's peak, with arms at the side and knees high. Softly land into the water in a standing position, using the water's resistance to cushion the impact.

You can perform multiple jumps in succession to build strength and endurance, utilizing the water's resistance for a safer, effective workout. The water's resistance reduces impact on the joints while increasing the workout intensity due to the effort required to move quickly against the water. This makes the moves particularly beneficial for enhancing strength, flexibility, cardiovascular fitness in a lower-impact, aquatic environment, that boosts your anaerobic and athletic power.

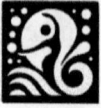

Questions for Reflection and Positive Action

1. **Performance Enhancement Reflection**: Reflect on how adding *Splash*Dance plyometrics into your training regimen can impact your athletic performance. What specific plyometric exercises would you like to try?

2. **Cross-Training Benefits**: How do you see the integration of water plyometrics benefiting your overall training strategy? How might you increase or modify water plyometrics to reach your desired training goals?

3. **Experiment with Variety**: Choose a new plyometric exercise from the list provided, such as Pikes or Air Jacks, and integrate it into your next training session. Afterward, analyze how the resistance of the water altered the intensity and effectiveness of the exercise compared to land-based plyometrics.

4. **Long-Term Athletic Goals**: Can you set a long-term goal related to athletic performance, such as improving power or agility? Outline a game plan for how you will use water plyometrics to achieve this goal over the next training season.

CHAPTER 22

Core Control and Abdominal Exercises in the Pool

Performing abdominal exercises in the pool is a superb way to target your core muscles, (the abdominals, back, side, buttock, and pelvic muscles), by utilizing the resistance and buoyancy of water. Maintaining proper form, focusing on core engagement, and adjusting the movements according to your fitness level are essential for effective results. This chapter delves deeper into various exercises that strengthen your core, both in standing positions and while buoyantly suspended in the water.

Comprehensive Benefits of Aquatic Abdominal Exercise Training

- **Core Strength:** Strengthens vital muscle groups including the abdominals: rectus abdominis, obliques, and transverse abdominis, as well the back muscles.

- **Balance and Stability:** Engages core muscles crucial for improving balance and stability in and out of water.

- **Low Impact:** Offers a cushioning exercise alternative, ideal for individuals with joint concerns or recovering from injuries.

Adding abdominal exercises into your pool workout not only diversifies your exercise regimen but also significantly enhances your abdominal and back strength. Whether you are a beginner or a seasoned athlete, these pool exercises offer a refreshing, effective, and enjoyable way to improve your fitness level. Embrace the challenge and soothing nature of aquatic abdominal exercises and transform your core strength.

Abdominal Conditioning Body Positions

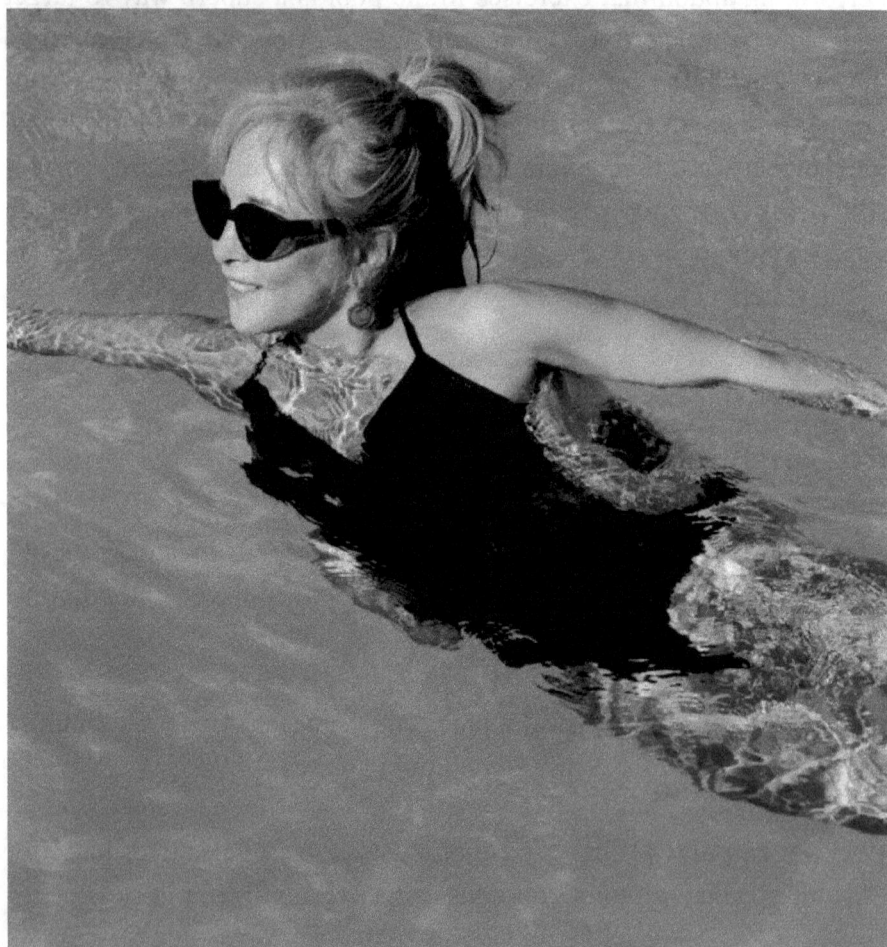

Photo: Lianna Tarantin

In abdominal and back conditioning exercises, selecting your appropriate body position is influenced by various factors, including your physical capabilities, comfort, the type of equipment used, and water depth, which can affect the feasibility of certain movements like standing crunches in waist-deep water. The most effective and comfortable positions for abdominal exercises generally include standing upright in chest-deep water at the shallow end of the pool with minimal hip and knee flexion. This position allows for the incorporation of buoyant equipment in front of your body to add resistance. Alternatively, exercises can also be performed vertically, diagonally, and horizontally in deeper water; this may require more skill and balance. Lying horizontally in a supine stance, using buoyancy aids, lets you focus on the moves while offering you safety and comfort. There are lots of ways to apply exercise modifications.

Key Focus on Form Concentrating on engaging your abdominal muscles is crucial throughout these exercises. Proper form ensures maximum effectiveness and helps you avoid injuries. Mindfully aim to concentrate and control the abdominal muscles effectively to achieve the desired results.

Types of Abdominal Exercises in the Pool

Abdominals-Standing in the Water:

1. **Standing Crunch (Aqua barbells):** Position your feet shoulder-width apart. Cradle aqua dumbells in front of you and perform a crunch by lowering your shoulders towards your hips, creating a "C" with your spine. This targets the core intensely.

2. **Standing Rotation (Aqua barbells):** With feet planted firmly, hold the aqua barbells close and rotate your torso side to side, engaging your core throughout the movement.

3. **Standing Modified Side Bends (Aqua barbells):** Stand tall, holding aqua barbells, and perform side bends. Keep your knees slightly bent and focus on engaging the oblique muscles.

Abdominals-Buoyant in the Water with a Floatation Belt or a Noodle Behind Your Back For Support:

1. **Recline Crunch:** Begin in a reclined position, legs extended. Perform a crunch by lifting your shoulders towards your knees, engaging your core.

2. **Recline Knee Tuck:** From the same reclined position, draw your knees towards your chest while lifting your shoulders, focusing on the lower insertion of the abdominal muscle group.

3. **Reverse Curl:** In a reclined position, lift your hips towards the surface, emphasizing the engagement of the lower insertion of the abdominals.

4. **Opposite Knee and Heel Reach:** Alternate reaching towards the opposite heels in front, and then behind you, enhancing oblique engagement.

5. **Side Lying Crunch:** From a side-lying position, perform crunches by lifting your shoulders towards your knees, focusing on lateral abdominal muscles.

6. **Facing the Noodle, Aqua Plank with Knee Tucks:** Get into a plank position with your forearms resting on a noodle and with your body in a straight line. Engage your core and lift one knee up towards your chest, then return it to the starting position. Alternate legs and repeat the movement. This exercise not only targets your abdominal muscles but also works your shoulders, chest, and back.

Aqua Abdominal Variations for Enhanced Challenges:

1. **Pendulum-Side:** Begin in a vertical position, using aqua barbells, or a noodle, for added resistance. Tuck your knees into your torso and lean your body to one side as the legs extend to the opposite side, engaging the core dynamically. You make keep your arms at the side, on the surface, in a "T" shape.

2. **Heel Diamond Crunch:** In a recline position, position your feet toward each other with knees apart, forming a diamond shape. Perform a crunch towards the center of the knees, intensifying the focus on the lower abdominals' insertion.

3. **Pelvic Tilt:** In a reclined position, emphasize your abdominal contractions as you pull your buttocks in, focusing on strong and controlled muscle engagement from chest to knees.

More Core Training for Abdominals and Back in the Pool

Embrace the unique challenge and soothing nature of these additional abdominal aquatic exercises:

1. **Water Crunches:** Stand in chest-deep water, either against the pool wall or using a pool noodle for support. Cross your arms over your chest and contract your abdominal muscles to curl your upper body forward, then slowly return to the starting position. This exercise targets your rectus abdominis muscles and strengthens your core.

2. **Flutter Kicks:** Hold onto the pool wall or a flotation device for support. Extend your legs straight and perform alternating up-and-down kicks. Keep your core engaged and maintain a steady rhythm to work the insertion of your lower abdominal muscles and to improve hip stability.

3. **Knee Tucks:** In waist-deep water, hold onto the pool wall or use a flotation device for support. Draw your knees up towards your chest, engaging your abdominal muscles, then slowly lower your legs back down. This movement focuses on the abdominals and hip flexors.

4. **Side Bends:** Stand in shoulder-deep water with your feet hip-width apart. Place one hand on your hip and extend the other hand overhead. Bend your torso to the side, focusing on engaging your oblique muscles, then return to the starting position and repeat on the other side. This exercise targets the obliques and enhances lateral core strength and stability.

5. **Sitting Twists:** Sit on a pool noodle or flotation device with your legs extended in front of you and your torso leaning back at a 45-degree angle. Rotate your torso from side to side, with your hands on each side. This exercise works the obliques and rectus abdominis and improves rotational core strength.

6. **One-Legged Bicycles** - Perform bicycle motions one leg at a time, emphasizing the feeling of peddling, your balance, and the exquisite rotation from the hip.

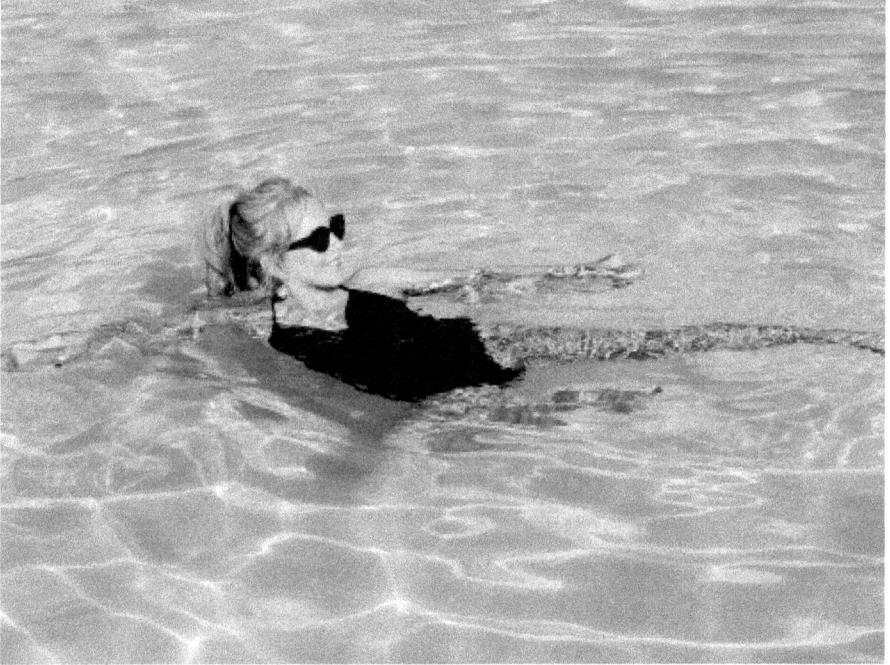

Photo: Lianna Tarantin

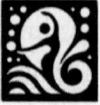

Questions for Reflection and Positive Action

1. **Abdominal Exercises in the Pool**: How do different abdominal exercises in the pool make you feel?

2. **Muscle Engagement Variations**: What differences do you notice in muscle engagement when performing standing versus buoyant abdominal exercises in the water?

3. **Balance and Stability Challenges**: In what ways can balance and stability challenges in the water improve your core training outcomes?

4. **Experiment with Body Positions**: Practice both standing and buoyant abdominal exercises. Note the differences in how the exercises feel. Which moves seem most effective for targeting different parts of your core?

5. **Incorporate Equipment**: Use aqua barbells or noodles during your next few workouts to vary resistance and challenge your muscles differently. How does this affect the intensity of your core exercises?

6. **Challenge Your Stability**: Intentionally incorporate exercises that challenge your stability, like the Side Lying Crunch or Reclined Oblique Twist and Tuck. Observe how these movements feel around your core strength and balance.

CHAPTER 23

Essential Elements Recap - Force, Intensity, Range of Motion & Alignment

Several key concepts, including force, intensity, range of motion, and alignment, are involved in aqua fitness training. Let's recap these important elements in the context of water-based exercises.

1. **Force:** In aqua fitness training, force refers to the amount of resistance encountered while performing exercises. Water provides natural resistance due to its density, which makes it an excellent medium for strength training. The force exerted against the body during movements helps to engage and strengthen muscles. By utilizing the resistance of water, you can work on improving your muscular strength and endurance.

2. **Intensity:** Intensity in aqua fitness training is related to the effort or level of exertion put into the exercises. It can be adjusted by modifying factors such as speed, resistance, and complexity of movements. Intensity is crucial for achieving fitness goals and can be tailored to accommodate different fitness levels. For example, high-intensity interval training (HIIT) can be implemented by alternating between periods of intense effort and active recovery. A lower intensity training protocol could involve water walking, gentle movement, and more relaxation.

3. **Range of Motion:** The range of motion refers to the extent to which a joint can be moved in a particular direction. Aqua fitness training allows for a greater range of motion compared to exercises performed on land due to the buoyancy and reduced impact on joints. Water provides support and reduces the effects of gravity, allowing you to move your joints through a wider range without placing excessive stress on the body. This can aid in improving flexibility, joint mobility, and overall functional movement.

4. **Alignment:** Proper alignment is essential in aqua fitness training to ensure optimal movement efficiency, reduce the risk of injury, and engage the correct muscles. Maintaining good alignment involves proper posture, core stability, and mindful body awareness while performing exercises in water. Aqua workouts incorporate movements in multiple directions; maintaining alignment helps to enhance the effectiveness of the exercise while minimizing stress on the body.

5. **Hydrostatic Pressure:** refers to the pressure exerted by water on the body when submerged. Hydrostatic pressure helps promote blood flow from the extremities back to the heart, enhancing circulation throughout the body. It supports and stabilizes joints, making movements smoother and less painful, which is beneficial for individuals with arthritis or injuries. Hydrostatic pressure plays a vital role in making *Splash*Dance effective for improving cardiovascular health and enhancing physical rehabilitation. Finally, the hydrostatic pressure exerted by the water can help reduce swelling, and provide gentle compression to the body, promoting recovery and reducing post-workout soreness.

The properties of water, such as its resistance, buoyancy, and hydrostatic pressure, contribute to the unique benefits of aqua fitness training. Water's resistance challenges the muscles throughout the entire range of motion, providing a comprehensive workout. Buoyancy reduces the impact on joints, making it a low-impact exercise option suitable for people with certain joint conditions or injuries.

The buoyancy of water enhances both flexibility and range of motion: while the hydrostatic pressure of water massages the working muscles.

Mindfully applying resistance is a fun and challenging way to train. You will actually feel a difference depending on how you "modify" the size, shape, and position of your body in the water.

At a Glance: Tips You Can Use To Increase (or Decrease) Your Training Intensity

Here is a recap, with tips to help you increase the intensity or benefits of your aqua fitness training. To reduce the intensity, <u>decrease</u> the following:

1. Increase the speed of movement (Law of Acceleration).

2. Increase the length of the lever.

3. Increase the range of motion of a specific joint.

4. Flex your extremities to implement the "eddy" resistance or drag forces.

5. Increase the width of your frontal plane.

6. Change directions often (Law of Action and Reaction)

7. Combine muscle groups- stride your legs to train the hamstrings and quadriceps while doing biceps curls with your arms to work your biceps and triceps.

*Splash*Dance includes a variety of training modalities, including water aerobics, intervals, circuits, rhythmic movements, water jogging, deep-water training, resistance training, aquatic equipment, abdominals, Tabata high intensity interval training (HIIT), relaxation and more.

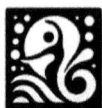

Questions for Reflection and Positive Action

1. **Personal Application of Concepts**: Reflect on how you currently apply the concepts of force, intensity, range of motion, and alignment in your aqua fitness routines. Are there any specific variations where you might be able to enhance your application of these concepts to improve your exercise effectiveness?

2. **Experiment with Intensity**: Experiment with adjusting the intensity of your aqua fitness training. You could try increasing the speed of your movements or changing the direction more frequently.

3. **Alignment Focus**: Which movements make maintaining proper alignment more challenging?

4. **Range of Motion Exploration**: Choose an exercise and perform it with varying ranges of motion—first

with a limited range, then with the maximum range your body comfortably allows. How does this change affect the difficulty of the movement and the muscles engaged?

5. **Force and Resistance Awareness**: Next time you are in the pool, consciously focus on the resistance provided by the water during different exercises. Experiment with altering your body position, such as changing the width of your frontal plane or flexing your extremities, to modify the resistance. How do these changes influence the overall challenge and benefit of the exercise.

CHAPTER 24

Training Stability Skills in *Splash*Dance

In the context of pool training, stability refers to the ability to maintain control and balance while performing exercises in the water. It involves having a solid and controlled body position in the water, and resisting instability caused by the dynamic nature of water and the forces exerted on the body. Here's why stability matters:

1. **Injury Prevention**: Having good stability in the water helps reduce the risk of injury during pool workouts. By maintaining control, balance, and mindful awareness, you can minimize the chances of slipping, falling, or sudden movements that could lead to strains, sprains, or other injuries. Stable movements also help protect your joints and muscles from excessive stress.

2. **Proper Technique**: Stability is closely related to proper technique and form in the water. When you have good stability, you can execute movements more effectively, and get the most out of your training. Stability allows you to maintain the correct alignment, engage the targeted muscles, and perform the desired movements with precision. This, in turn, improves your training effectiveness and helps you achieve your fitness goals more efficiently.

3. **Core Activation and Strength**: Stability in the pool heavily relies on core activation and strength. Your core muscles, including the abdominals, obliques, and back muscles, play a crucial role in stabilizing your body during water exercises. Training for stabil-

ity leads to overall functional strength. A strong core enhances your ability to perform various movements, (including activities of daily living), maintain balance, and transfer power effectively through the body.

4. **Balance and Proprioception**: Aqua Fitness training provides an environment where balance and proprioception (the body's sense of its position in space) are constantly challenged. Water's buoyancy and resistance require constant adjustments and control to maintain balance. Working on stability in the pool helps improve your balance and proprioceptive abilities, both in water and on land. These enhanced skills can benefit your overall co-ordination, posture, stability, and performance in various daily activities and sports.

5. **Experiment with Props:** It's fun to "gamify," and play with props you might have on hand. These might include frisbees, 2-5-pound light hand weights, canes, kick boards, or noodles that challenge your stability and resistance.

6. **Rehabilitation and Recovery:** If you are recovering from an injury or managing certain challenges, pool training with an emphasis on safety and stability can be truly beneficial. The water's buoyancy reduces the impact and stress on joints, allowing for a gentler rehabilitation environment. Stability training helps rebuild strength, ROM, and neuromuscular control, aiding in the recovery process.

Enhancing Stability in *Splash*Dance: Mastering Aquatic Equipment and Balance

Using aquatic equipment in *Splash*Dance introduces a dynamic challenge that necessitates increased stabilization and kinesthetic awareness in order to target balance, core strength, and control. In order to maintain essential proper posture, avoid leaning forward—remember, the buoyancy will support your rear.

Practices such as standing on one leg, balancing on pool noodles, and executing controlled movements with both arms and legs are pivotal. Additionally, employing specialized aquatic equipment, aqua barbells, floatation belts, noodles, can significantly improve your ability to manage and adapt to the water's resistance, leading to a stronger, more balanced body. Embrace these techniques to refine your stability and enjoy a safer, more effective *Splash*Dance experience.

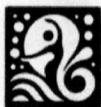

Questions for Reflection and Positive Action

1. **Personal Stability Assessment**: Reflect on your current level of stability during your aqua training. What are some movements or exercises that help improve your stability, and enhance your overall performance and safety?

2. **Core Activation Focus**: During your next pool session, consciously focus on engaging your core muscles throughout various exercises. Note any differences in your stability and control. How did it feel?

3. **Balance Improvement Plan**: Why not create a game plan to improve your balance and proprioception by mindfully maintaining control in water's dynamically unstable condition. How will you celebrate your progress?

4. **Recovery and Rehabilitation Connection**: If it applies, consider any past injuries or recovery processes you've experienced. How could focusing on stability in the pool aid in your rehabilitation and recovery, or help prevent future injuries?

CHAPTER 25

Monitoring, Adjusting, and Tuning Into Your Water Exercise Intensity

While water exercise may seem effortless, it actually requires significant muscular effort due to the resistance of the water. Sustained, vigorous movement with great form, considering duration, frequency, and varying intensities, are key to aqua fitness.

"To optimize your heart health and maximize cardiovascular benefits, aim to keep your heart rate in the sweet spot—between 60% and 85% of its maximum. This targeted zone ensures you harness the full power of your workout, efficiently boosting your heart's strength without pushing into the red zone. Stay in tune with your body's cues to maximize benefits and minimize risks.

Understanding Rate of Perceived Exertion (RPE)

Rate of Perceived Exertion is a subjective scale used to measure your perception of the intensity of your physical activity. Understanding your Rate of Perceived Exertion is key to adjecting your training intensity, based on how you feel during exercise. Here's why RPE is invaluable in aqua monitoring:

1. **Individualized Intensity**: RPE tailors your workout challenges based on your personal capability, goals, and desired outcomes.

2. **Adjustable Intensity**: RPE allows you to adapt to the water conditions and your personal energy levels, allowing for modifications on the fly.

3. **Body Awareness**: RPE enhances awareness of physical state and exertion, encouraging you to adjust for your comfort and challenge.

4. **Safety**: RPE helps prevent overexertion and keeps you safe.

5. **Progress Tracking**: RPE facilitates goal setting and monitoring fitness levels.

6. **Exercise Selection Flexibility**: RPE assists you in choosing exercises that match your desired intensity, challenges, and performance.

Familiarize yourself with the Borg Scale, which ranges from 6 to 20 to consistently assess your effort levels.

The Borg Scale and Rate of Perceived Exertion (RPE) in Aqua Fitness

What is Rate of Perceived Exertion (RPE): "Fine Tune" Your Training Intensity?

Rate of Perceived Exertion (RPE) provides a way to assess how hard or easy, you feel you are working during exercise. RPE is good to know, helpful in tuning in to your training, and recommended in an aqua fitness workout for several reasons:

1. **Individualized Intensity**: RPE allows you to gauge the intensity of your training based on your personal perception rather than relying solely on external factors like heart rate or speed. Since everyone's fitness level is different, RPE helps customize the intensity to suit your individual capabilities.

2. **Adjusting Intensity**: Aqua fitness workouts can vary in intensity based on factors such as water depth, speed, and exercise selection. By using RPE, you can modify the intensity of your workout to meet your specific goals. For example, you can increase or decrease the effort level based on your desired level of challenge, fitness level, or energy level on a given day.

3. **Listening to Your Body**: RPE encourages you to listen to your body and be aware of how you feel during exercise. It allows you to tune in to your physical sensations and adjust accordingly. If you feel fatigued or need to push harder, RPE provides a subjective measure to guide your effort level.

4. **Safety and Injury Prevention**: RPE is a useful tool for preventing overexertion and potential injuries during aqua fitness workouts. The water environment can sometimes mask feelings of fatigue or strain, making it important to rely on internal cues to gauge effort. RPE helps ensure safe and effective training.

5. **Goal Setting and Progress Tracking:** RPE can be used to set goals and track your progress. By comparing your RPE values, you can assess improvements in your fitness level. For instance, if you previously found a particular exercise to be very challenging (high RPE), but now perceive it as less demanding (lower RPE), it indicates progress and increasing fitness. Good on you.

6. **Flexibility in Exercise Selection**: RPE allows you to choose from a wide range of movements and exercises that align with your desired intensity level. For example, if you want a higher-intensity workout, you can select exercises that require more effort and generate a higher RPE.

It's important to note that in the water your heart rate may not accurately reflect your overall exercise intensity. If the water is cool, your heart rate may be artificially low. It may also be lower if you're in deeper water because of the pressure on your chest. So, in addition to periodically monitoring your heart rate, pay attention to how you feel. This is probably even more important. The Borg Scale offers a more accurate gauge of exertion by focusing on muscular fatigue and breath control.

Familiarize yourself with the Borg Rate of Perceived Exertion scale. Are your muscles tired? Can you utter a full sentence? Are you singing through a whole song? These are all clues to how intensely you are training. For maximum aerobic benefits, it's important to challenge yourself, know your body, and build progression, so you can leave your training feeling great, and wanting more!

Borg's Rating of Perceived Exertion (RPE) Scale	
Perceived Exertion Rating	**Description of Exertion**
6	No exertion; sitting and resting
7	Extremely light
8	
9	Very light
10	
11	Light
12	
13	Somewhat hard
14	
15	Hard
16	
17	Very hard
18	
19	Extremely hard
20	Maximal exertion

Borg, 1982

Aquatics Exercise Association founder, Ruth Sova says, "Many variables can affect the heart rate during aquatic exercise that it is impossible to depend on taking (traditional carotid and radial land working) heart rates as an indicator of intensity."

Borg's Rate of Perceived Exertion, and the Talk Test are better measures because of those variables. These methods allow you to listen to your body and genuinely access your training intensity, allowing you to maintain, gear up or down.

What is the Talk Test?

In the context of *Splash*Dance, or any fitness activity, the "talk test" is a simple and practical method to measure exercise intensity based on how easily you can talk while training. Here's a brief description:

The Talk Test: A Simple and Mindful Intensity Measure

The "talk test" is an easy, no-equipment-needed method to measure exercise intensity:

- **Light Intensity**: Full conversations are possible without any strain. You can sing through the song.

- **Moderate Intensity**: Talking is possible, but singing is not. Your breathing is deeper, requiring occasional pauses.

- **Vigorous Intensity**: Only short phrases or words are possible between breaths, suitable for shorter durations.

Ideally and depending on your goals, it's probably best to build progression and train in the moderate and vigorous intensity modes, depending on your desired outcomes.

"Working Heart Rates" Might Be Lower During *Splash*Dance

Though we recommend RPE, the Borg Scale and the Talk Test, it's good to know that physiological factors cause lower heart rates in water. Here's why:

1. **Buoyancy and Reduced Weight-Bearing**: There's less strain on the cardiovascular system due to reduced gravitational force.

2. **Hydrostatic Pressure**: Assists blood flow back to the heart, lessening the heart's workload.

3. **Cooling Effect**: Efficient heat dispersion through water reduces the need for the heart to pump vigorously.

4. **Muscle Relaxation and Vasodilation**: Relaxed muscles and dilated blood vessels lower cardiovascular demand.

5. **Training Adaptations**: Regular aquatic exercise enhances cardiac efficiency, lowering the required heart rate for the same exercise intensity. Your heart at rest becomes stronger over time with dedicated training.

In conclusion, utilizing tools such as the Talk Test, the Borg Scale, and the Rate of Perceived Exertion (RPE) offer a more practical and effective approach to monitoring exercise intensity during water workouts than measuring heart rate. These methods enable you to set realistic and optimal intensity levels, ensuring that each session is safe yet maximally beneficial. It's important to note that while the perceived effort in water might feel less intense due to the buoyancy and cooling effects, the cardiovascular benefits of your *Splash*Dance workout are substantial. By understanding and applying these perceptual scales, you can confidently navigate the intensity of your aquatic exercises, making every water session both enjoyable and efficacious.

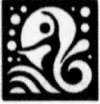

Questions for Reflection and Positive Action

1. **Experimenting with RPE**: During your next few water exercise sessions, use the Borg Scale to gauge your Rate of Perceived Exertion (RPE), and challenge yourself to meet your fitness and performance goals and needs.

2. **Application of the Talk Test**: Apply the "talk test" during your next workout session to assess its practicality and accuracy. Can you hold a conversation, or are you only able to speak in short phrases? How does this align with your perceived exertion level and training goals?

CHAPTER 26

Enhance Your Experience with Aquatic Resistance Equipment

A World of Aquatic Resistance Equipment

Incorporating resistance equipment into your *Splash*Dance regimen elevates the effectiveness of your water workouts by intensifying the resistance encountered during exercises. This chapter delves into a variety of tools and props that can enrich and intensify your aquatic exercise sessions, making them both more challenging and fun.

Use Your Noodle: An aqua "noodle" is a flexible, buoyant foam cylinder that is a versatile exercise tool. Here are some benefits, and ways to use your noodles.

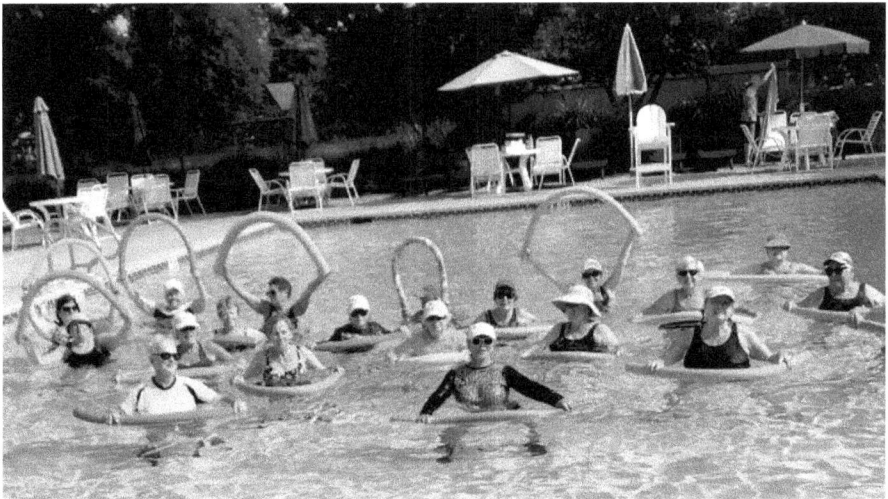

Photo at Fairway Mews, Spring Lake Heights.NJ

Benefits of Training With Aqua Noodles

1. **Buoyancy Support**: Noodles provide support in the water, making it easier for you to maintain your balance and stability.

2. **Resistance**: The water provides natural resistance, and using a noodle increases this resistance due to its surface area. This helps in strengthening muscles, challenging balance, and improving cardiovascular fitness.

3. **Versatility**: Noodles can be used for a variety of exercises targeting different body parts, including arms, legs, the core, and as a partner exercise.

4. **Low Impact**: Noodles' buoyancy reduces the impact on joints, making them an excellent rehabilitation option.

5. **Fun**: Noodles add an element of fun and variety to water workouts, helping to keep you engaged, motivated, and have fun cross-training in the pool.

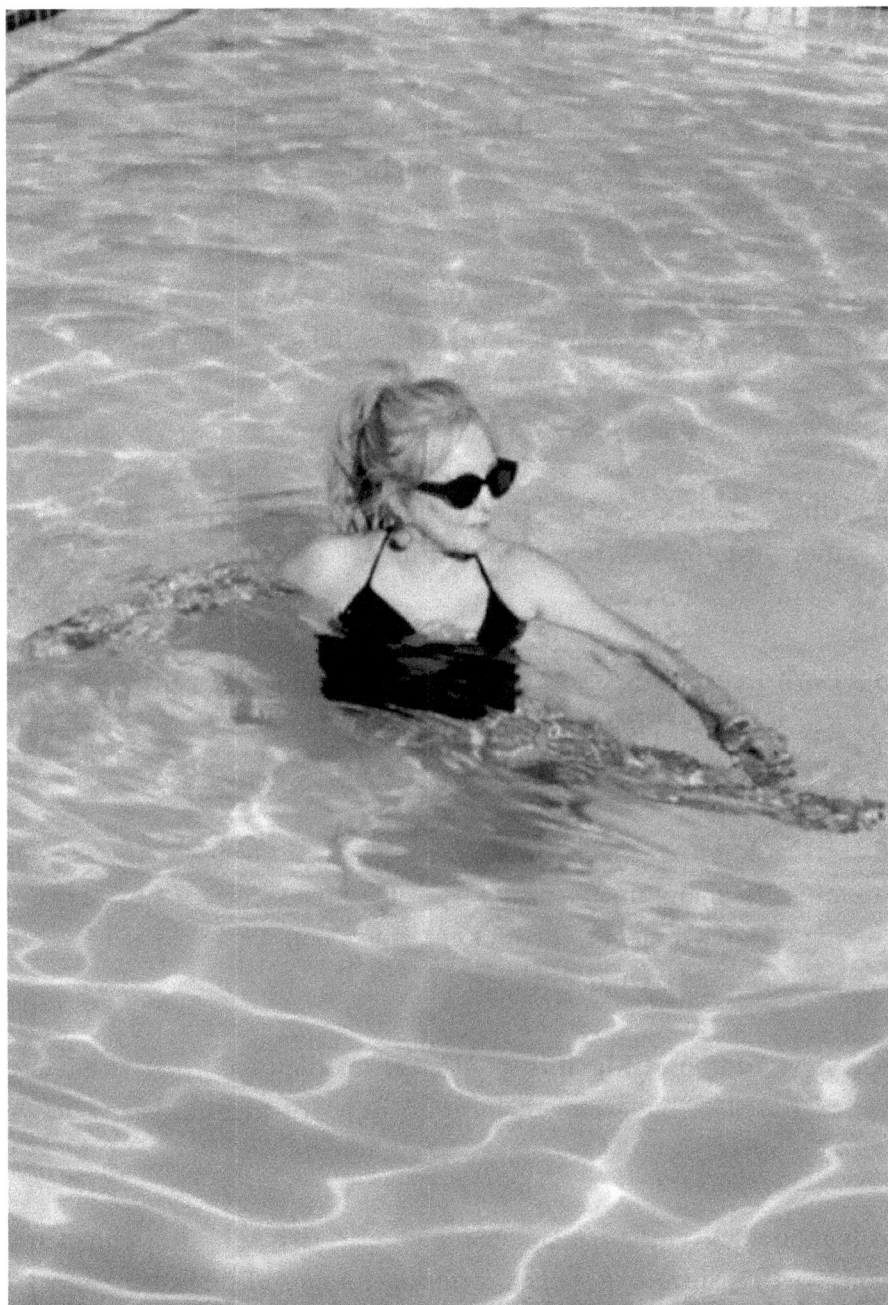

Photo: Lianna Tarantin

Ways to Use Aqua Noodles

1. **Alternating Leg Kicks:** Place the noodle behind your back. Reach your opposite hand toward your opposite leg, alternate, and continue. Try this standing or suspended in the water.

2. **Leg Exercises**: Place the noodle between your legs and use it for resistance as you perform kicks under water. This can help strengthen leg muscles and improve lower body endurance. Ride it like a horse.

3. **Upper Body Exercises**: Hold the noodle with both hands and push it down into the water, then pull it back up. This works the arms, shoulders, and chest.

4. **Core Exercises**: Sit on the noodle like a bicycle and pedal your legs while keeping your balance. Scull your hands and arms. This engages the core muscles effectively.

5. **Aqua Jogging**: Place the noodle under your arms or around your waist to maintain an upright position in deeper water, perform jogging movements, locomotion, and deep-water running. It's a great cardiovascular workout.

6. **Stretching and Flexibility**: Use the noodle to assist in stretching exercises in the water, helping to improve flexibility and range of motion.

Aqua noodles are an adaptable and effective tool for enhancing your *Splash*Dance experience, offering mind and body benefits and enjoyable exercise.

1. Aqua and Dumbells:

Constructed from buoyant materials like foam or plastic, these aqua barbells intensify upper body training. Exercises like bicep curls, shoulder presses, and triceps extensions become more challenging as you push and pull through the water's natural resistance.

2. Aquatic Resistance Bands:

These stretchable bands are tailored for water use, adding resistance to movements. Wrap them around your ankles, thighs, or upper body to perform exercises like leg kicks, lateral walks, or rowing motions, enhancing muscle engagement through the band's tension. These are not recommended if you suffer from high blood pressure.

3. Aqua Jogging Belts:

Designed to aid vertical movements such as jogging, high knees, kicking, or deep-water running, these buoyant belts help you stay afloat as you aim to maintain an upright position. Dynamic deep-water exercises with a belt are a great challenge and a benefit for your cardiovascular system.

4. Light Hand Weights:

While not traditionally aquatic, light hand weights (2-5 pounds) used in shallow water sessions enhance strength training by providing added resistance. These hand weights provide a challenge and are helpful in providing muscular strength and endurance. I love using light hand weights in the water to boost energy, endurance, and effort. It feels great.

5. Aqua Gloves:

These webbed gloves increase the surface area of your hands, boosting resistance as you move through the water, and are ideal for various exercises, including different swimming strokes and arm movements.

Incorporating Aqua Resistance Gloves Can Transform Your Training

Consider these surprising benefits to wearing aqua gloves:

- **Move Water, Get Stronger** – Encouraging you beyond 'going through the motions,' and "bouncing from move to move," wearing gloves makes your hands weblike, increasing surface area. Gloves powerfully increase resistance, getting your arms, shoulders, and chest stronger in less time.

- **Protect Your Joints**—In addition to increasing muscular strength and tone, wearing gloves inhibits movement, meaning you'll automatically avoid quick, jarring motions that might place unnecessary stress on the shoulders and elbows. Gloved hands in aqua aerobics can soothe joints by keeping your hands warm, too.

- **Greater Stretch and Cardio Potential** – You get a unique kind of stretch when your gloved hands are fluid and relaxed in moving against the water. Wearing gloves can gently pull the fingers forward and back for a feel-good muscle-lengthening water-assisted stretch. Further they boost your cardiovascular endurance in water running, cross-country skiing and other aerobic exercises.

- **Core Control** - When you wear gloves in water, movement becomes slower and requires greater control. This lets you target, and fire up your midsection in every movement, making every exercise a core exercise.

- **Improve Your Bone Health** - Wearing gloves helps increase your effort and supports strong, healthy bones. Over time you can play with ways of moving your hands and body in the water that offer you the resistance you desire.

Innovative Equipment and Pool Toys

Besides standard tools, innovative equipment like the Kona Aquatoner, fitness paddles, kickboards, fins or even homemade items like empty milk jugs can add fun and variety to your pool workouts. These "pool toys" encourage playful yet effective exercise, enhancing both enjoyment and positive fitness outcomes. You can use balls, balloons, and frisbees to add some fun to the mix. What can you play with in the pool?

Using resistance equipment leads to increased muscle engagement, strength building, and overall fitness gains. It's important to use the equipment properly and follow any instructions or guidelines provided by the manufacturer. You can gain cardiovascular endurance and muscular strength without equipment, but using equipment may increase the benefits of your aqua training.

Safety and Effectiveness Matters When Using Aqua Equipment

Focusing on your kinesthetic awareness in water is vital; avoid leaning too far forward or shrugging your shoulders continuously. Integrating balance and stability-focused exercises enhance your control and safety in the water.

Utilizing aquatic resistance equipment not only elevates the intensity of your water exercise but also broadens the scope of your *Splash*Dance training possibilities. From building muscle strength and endurance to improving cardiovascular health and joint protection, equipment can offer a far-reaching approach to enhancing your aquatic fitness journey.

More Fun Facts About Water and Aqua Gloves

Water is twelve times more resistant than air, and it offers you the opportunity for a positive training effect in a variety of wonderful ways as we have discussed. I enjoy wearing gloves in order to increase my hands surface area, and for the extra resistance that they offer. You can really feel it when you can actively push and pull, gloved, against the water.

Swim gloves look and fit like a glove, but the webbing between each finger helps grab and resist the water with each stroke. Aqua gloves help to protect the joints, encourage building your cardiovascular power, and move you to being a stronger, vibrant, and more flexible you. When you know how to use the water it becomes the ultimate training tool.

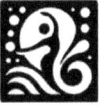

Questions for Reflection and Positive Action

1. **Equipment Exploration**: Reflect on the various types of aquatic resistance equipment described. Which type of equipment are you most interested in trying out, and why? Plan a fun session where you incorporate various equipment into your routine.

2. **Personal Adaptation**: Consider your current fitness goals and the resistance equipment available to you. How could integrating specific tools, like aqua gloves or floatation belt, better help you achieve these goals?

3. **Safety and Technique**: Choose one or two pieces of equipment and focus on mastering their use while maintaining proper form and alignment.

4. **Circuit Training**: Set up a circuit with different equipment and non-equipment stations. What could you include to boost the fun factor and your training?

CHAPTER 27

Tabata or High Intensity Interval Training (HIIT)

Tabata training in the pool is a high-intensity interval training (HIIT) workout adapted for an aquatic environment. The Tabata protocol, developed by Dr. Izumi Tabata, involves exercises performed in short bursts of intense effort followed by brief rest periods. Here's how Tabata training translates to the pool setting:

Structure of Tabata Training in the Pool:

- **Duration**: Each Tabata session typically lasts about 4 minutes. It consists of 8 rounds of 20 seconds of intense exercise followed by 10 seconds of rest.

- **Intensity**: The exercises are performed at a high intensity, leveraging the water's resistance to increase the workout's challenge without the high impact of similar land-based exercises.

- **Exercises**: Activities can vary from aqua jogging, tuck jumps, and cross-country skiing motions, to other dynamic movements like flutter kicks, pool planks, or even resistance moves using aqua barbells or noodles.

Benefits of Tabata Training in the Pool:

Efficient Cardio Workout: Due to its high intensity, Tabata can provide significant cardiovascular benefits in a shorter period.

Low Impact: The buoyancy of the water reduces the impact on joints, making it suitable for those with joint issues or those recovering from injuries.

Calorie Burning: High-intensity intervals can lead to higher calorie burn during and after the workout due to the increased metabolic rate.

Versatility: Exercises can be varied widely, which helps maintain engagement and prevents boredom.

Strengthens Muscles: The resistance of the water enhances muscle strengthening and endurance without the need for heavy weights.

Incorporating Tabata training into aquatic exercise routines can be a powerful way to enhance your fitness level. It also offers a fun and challenging variation whereby Tabata training truly capitalizes on the unique properties of water.

Interval Training in Aquatic Fitness Review: Interval training in a pool is a dynamic and efficient method to enhance your *Splash*Dance experience. By alternating between high-intensity bursts and lower-intensity recovery periods, this training approach offers a balanced workout that maximizes both effort and recovery. Here's how incorporating interval training can transform your aqua fitness regime:

Aqua Interval Training, and Tabata: High Intensity Interval Training (HIIT) Benefits

1. Boosts Your Cardiovascular Fitness:
High-intensity intervals elevate your heart rate, significantly enhancing cardiovascular endurance.

Continuous challenges to your heart and lungs improve their efficiency, increasing your overall aerobic capacity and cardiovascular health.

2. Enhanced Calorie Burning and Weight Loss:
Interval training accelerates your heart rate during high-intensity bursts, leading to increased calorie burn.

The unique cycle of intense activity followed by recovery periods keeps your metabolism elevated, helping you burn more calories during and after the workout, and promoting effective weight loss.

3. Increased Muscle Endurance and Strength:
Engaging multiple muscle groups, high-intensity intervals in the pool use the resistance of water to intensify the workout.

This strengthens muscles across your arms, shoulders, core, and legs, and also builds endurance, enabling you to perform better and longer.

4. Mental Stimulation and Workout Variety:
Interval training introduces a diverse array of exercises, such as aqua jogging, kicks, deep-water running, skipping and other high-intensity water aerobics, keeping the routine engaging and mentally stimulating.

This variety helps in maintaining high motivation levels and prevents the monotony often associated with fitness routines.

5. Joint-Friendly, Low-Impact Workouts:
The buoyancy of water cushions joints, making interval training ideal for those with joint concerns, arthritis, or post-injury recovery needs.

Despite its high intensity, the aquatic environment minimizes the risk of joint impact injuries, offering a safe platform for vigorous exercise.

6. Time Efficiency:
Interval training is particularly valued for its ability to deliver significant fitness benefits in a condensed time frame.

This efficiency makes it perfect for those with busy schedules, enabling you to achieve more with shorter workouts.

Implementing Interval Training in Your Routine

To effectively integrate interval training into your pool workouts, consider:

Tailored Intervals: Customize the duration and intensity of the intervals according to your current fitness level and specific training goals.

A Progressive Challenge: As your endurance and strength improve, gradually increase both the intensity and length of the high-intensity periods to continuously challenge your body and advance your fitness.

Balanced Approach: Always start with a thorough warm-up to prepare the body for high-intensity work and conclude with a cool-down period to safely bring the heart rate back to normal, followed by a final stretch and relaxation.

When incorporating intervals into your pool training program, it's essential to structure your intervals based on your fitness level, goals, and the specific exercises you choose. Gradually increase the intensity and duration of your intervals over time to continue challenging your body and progressing your fitness.

Interval training in a pool setting like *Splash*Dance offers a multi-faceted approach to fitness that combines the physical benefits of intense exercise with the therapeutic qualities of water. By adopting interval training, you can enjoy a holistic workout that promotes cardiovascular health, muscle development, and weight management, all while protecting your joints and keeping your training engaging and manageable within your busy lifestyle.

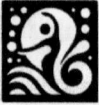

Questions for Reflection and Positive Action

1. **Personal Experience with Tabata**: Reflect on your first experience with Tabata training in the pool. How did the high intensity and short duration of the intervals affect your perception of effort and overall endurance? What did you find most challenging and rewarding about this training method?

2. **Adjusting Interval Intensity**: Based on your current fitness level, how might you adjust the intensity and duration of the Tabata intervals to better suit your needs? Plan a session where you experiment with these adjustments, noting any differences in how you feel during and after the workout.

3. **Exercise Selection for Tabata**: Consider the variety of exercises you can incorporate into your Tabata sessions. Choose two or three new movements to include in your next session and assess their impact on your workout intensity and enjoyment.

4. **Long-Term Planning**: How could regular Tabata training in the pool influence your long-term fitness goals?

CHAPTER 28

Sound Waves - *Splash*Dance Rhythms and Your Pitch Perfect Playlist

"Music is like water. It is something that must flow.
Music flows from one heart to another."

- Jiddu Krishnamurti, Indian Philosopher, Writer, and Spiritual Figure.

Music, melodies, and rhythms can activate, motivate, energize, comfort, relax, and connect us. Being "moved" by music is a global and ancient tradition. Focusing on the synergy between sound, rhythm, and physical movement in water, music plays an essential role in enhancing the *Splash*Dance experience. A moving musical selection can motivate you, guide the pace of your training, and enhance your overall performance. The artful curation of music enhances and elevates the flow and energy of the aqua fitness experience.

Rhythmic Depths: The Power of Music in Aqua Fitness

Revel in the world of music! Music's motivational power transcends mere beats per minute. It's about the "feeling" carried by the rhythms, which is especially palpable when you are moving through the water. Whether you're gliding smoothly or pushing against the current, the right music can infuse elements of energy, strength, power or even tranquility into your routine. Encouraging creativity in both choreography and musical selection, *Splash*Dance champions the use of inspiring, enjoyable tunes to elevate the mood and effectiveness of each and every aqua training session.

Crafting Your Pitch Perfect, Strategic Playlist

Creating a playlist for *Splash*Dance goes beyond simply selecting background music; it involves making strategic choices that profoundly enhance your workout experience. Music serves as a dynamic motivator, naturally prompting rhythmic and synchronized movements. A well-constructed playlist is not just a sequence of songs but a journey that adjusts the atmosphere, pace, and intensity of your session. It effectively guides you through varying energy levels—starting with invigorating warm-ups, moving through vigorous high-intensity intervals and aerobic sequences, progressing into strength, and toning exercises, and finally easing into stretching, conditioning, and a calming cooldown. Each track is carefully chosen to ensure that it supports and enriches every phase of your aqua fitness routine, making each workout both challenging and enjoyable.

Explore a World of Music

Music is not just motivating; it's a crucial element that enhances your enjoyment and commitment to exercise. With a vast world of musical styles at your fingertips, each genre holds the potential to amplify the flow, enjoyment, and fun of your workouts. Dive into this diverse musical landscape to discover the perfect tracks that elevate your *SplashDance* experience and keep you coming back for more.

Explore and Enjoy Across a Diverse Array of Musical Genres including: Alternative Avant -Garde, Big Band, Bluegrass, Breaking/

Scratching, Hymns, Classical, Orchestrated Band, Comedy, Contemporary, Country—Western, Disco, Easy Listening, Folk, Fusion free form jazz, Gospel, Holiday, Instrumental, Jazz, Latin-American, Meditation, New Age, Movie Soundtracks, Neoclassical, New Wave, Era of your choice, Reggae, Ragtime, Rhythm and Blues, Rock and Roll, Soul Synthesized, Theme Songs, Holidays and Celebrations, Top Forty, Funk

Diverse Musical Genres

*Splash*Dance celebrates a variety of musical styles, themes, and rhythms to respect diverse tastes and to match music to the desired outcome of the training mode. Why not try:

- Pop and Rock for high-energy routines

- Classical and Big Band for structured movements

- Latin and Caribbean tunes for rhythmic and dance-inspired sessions

- Songs you enjoyed when you were growing up or celebrating a peak moment.

- Special themed music around celebrations, holidays, and traditions.

Creating Effective Playlists

- **Sequencing:** Arrange music to gradually build intensity and then taper off. Start with upbeat tracks to warm up, use steady rhythms for the main session, and slow down the tempo for cooldowns, and gentle stretching.

- **Variety:** Include a mix of genres and tempos to keep you engaged, and moving through different energy levels, workout phases, and with enjoyment.

Utilizing Music for Choreography

- **Predictive Planning:** Use the beat and rhythm of the music to plan and synchronize movements so that they match the musical phrasing.

- **Motivational Cues:** Select music with motivational lyrics or rhythms that encourage you to push through challenging segments.

Adapting Music to Your Needs

- **Personalization:** Choose music that resonates with you, and your preferences. This personal touch can significantly enhance your positive engagement.

- **Appropriate Tempo:** Choose music that supports the intended intensity of the exercise without encouraging overly rapid movements that could lead to injury or frustration.

- **Lyrics and Mood:** Ensure that the music's lyrics are appropriate and uplifting, contributing positively to the training environment and experience.

Sample Playlist for *Splash*Dance Aqua Fitness

Warm-Up:

- **"Levitating"** by Dua Lipa – Energizing. Sets the pace to prepare you physically and mentally by increasing heart rate and circulation.

- **"Firework"** by Katy Perry - a dance, pop, self-empowerment song with inspirational lyrics.

- **"Hooked on Classics"** by Louis Clark and the London Philharmonic Symphony – A powerful, familiar, and fun classical piece that inspires positive movement at the get go. Great to warm up if the pool is chilly.

- **"Sweet Freedom"** by Michael MacDonald – a soulful and long piece of music with great variation for a warmup, stretch, and light intervals.

Aerobic Section

- **"Uptown Funk"** by Mark Ronson and Bruno Mars - This funky, high-energy track is perfect for getting you moving with its catchy beat and vibrant brass sections.

- **"Happy"** by Pharrell Williams - It's infectious rhythm and joyful lyrics make it an excellent choice for creating a positive and uplifting mood.

- **"Shake It Off" by Taylor Swift** - This pop anthem with its bouncy beats is great for high-intensity dance moves, encouraging everyone to shake off their worries and any distress.

- **"Walking on Sunshine" by Katrina and the Waves** - An enduring feel-good song that's all about feeling great and energetic, ideal for a mid-session pick-me-up. Great for deep-water running, and intervals.

- **Don't Start Now"** by Dua Lipa – High tempo, nice for high-intensity intervals.

Strengthening, Toning, Conditioning

- **"Ain't No Mountain High Enough"** by Marvin Gaye and Tammi Terrell - The powerful vocals and uplifting tempo make this song ideal for maintaining energy during strength exercises.

- **"Isn't She Lovely"** by Stevie Wonder - The lovely steady beat provides a great rhythm for exercises that require controlled movements and core engagement.

- **"Reach Out I'll Be There"** by The Four Tops - The driving beat and emotional intensity can help motivate participants to push through more challenging toning and strengthening routines.

Cool Down: Calm, Soothing Melodies Support Relaxation and Recovery

- **"Golden Hour"** by Kygo & Whitney Houston – Smooth and calming, ideal for stretching and relaxation.

- **"Ocean Eyes"** by Billie Eilish – Soothing, perfect for final relaxation and mindfulness.

- **"Solar Power"** by Lorde - for cooldowns, aiding in relaxation and calm.

- **"La Isla Bonita"** – Madonna – Melodic and lovely, slow rhythms

Relaxation

- **"Sailing"** by Christopher Cross – Calming, slow and easy; perfect for breathing a slow "Breath of Thanks."

- **"Caribbean Blue"** by Enya – Song inspires cooling down and stretching,

Choosing and curating music for aqua fitness programs like *Splash*-Dance requires a nuanced understanding of how music, movement, and mood interact. By thoughtfully selecting and sequencing music, you can significantly enhance the effectiveness of your training. The goal is to create an auditory environment that not only complements the physical activities but also enriches the overall fitness experience, creating a fun and supportive atmosphere that benefits both individuals and in a group, the community.

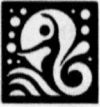

Questions for Reflection and Positive Action

1. **Personal Music Influence**: Reflect on how different types of music influence your mood and energy levels. Can you identify music that motivates, and moves you?

2. **Playlist Customization**: Create a customized playlist for your *Splash*Dance session, considering the program structure from warm-up to cooldown, to final stretch. What songs and types of music would you like to include?

3. **Exploring Genres**: Experiment with incorporating different genres of music you typically wouldn't use. For example, if you usually rely on pop or rock, try adding a few classical or country tracks. Note any differences in how these genres influence engagement, enjoyment, and the dynamics.

CHAPTER 29

Sample Format - *Splash*Dance Safety, Effectiveness & FUN!

From tiny, tiny waves of joy, one gets to the ocean
of happiness, which is called bliss.

— *Maharishi Mahesh Yogi, the Creator of Transcendental Meditation*

When designing an effective and enjoyable Aqua-powered fitness program, it's essential to consider the exercise guidelines set by the American College of Sports Medicine. These professional standards also address specific goals, needs, and safety guidelines.

The American College of Sports Medicine (ACSM) Guidelines for Aerobic Fitness

We recommend following the ACSM guidelines for aerobic fitness, which offer the following recommendations:

Frequency	Duration	Intensity
3 to 5 days a week	20 to 60 minutes	55% to 90% of estimated maximum heart rate

The ACSM additionally recommends a minimum of two total-body strength sessions a week. It's exciting to note that the *Splash*Dance protocol combines aerobics, strength, and flexibility training, and more to help you reach your ACSM goals.

Key Considerations for Designing and Customizing Your _Splash_Dance Experience:

Depth and Pool Shape: Adapt exercises to accommodate the water depth and the geometric layout of the pool.

Bottom Surface: Assess the pool floor for smoothness and note any changes in depth to avoid injuries. In any case, it's recommended to wear footwear.

Temperature and Available Equipment: Adjust the intensity of activities to suit the water temperature and add available equipment to enhance your exercise effectiveness, complexity, and variety.

Edge and Deck Surface: Ensure safety by considering the pool edge and the surrounding deck area, especially in terms of slip resistance.

Fun Formula – Playing at the Pool's Edge

If your pool design permits, use the pool's edge creatively for interval, core, or flexibility training. Following a cardiovascular segment, the edge can be employed for exercises like side bends or mountain climbers, adding variety to the routine. Cheerleader jumps, with hands on the deck, and lifting up out of the pool, offer an aerobic burst of energy. Longer lingering stretches at the wall are worth savoring.

Sample Class Structure:

1. **Warmup (5-10 minutes)**: Start with rhythmical movements to gently elevate your body's temperature. Initially use short levers and then progress to longer levers. The warm up increases blood

flow to your muscles while releasing synovial fluid in the joints for better mobility and range of motion. Warmups incorporate static stretching, and light, easy movement to prepare the respiratory, cardiovascular, and muscular systems for the increased activity.

2. **Cardiovascular Conditioning (25-35 minutes)**: With the body adequately warmed up, increase the workout intensity to remain within your target zone, adhering to ACSM guidelines (50% - 85% of heart rate reserve, The Borg Rate of Perceived Exertion (RPE) levels of "somewhat hard" to "hard"), or the Talk Test. This segment not only enhances aerobic capacity but also builds muscle strength and endurance, particularly for the legs and upper body.

3. **Muscular Strength and Aqua Abdominal Conditioning (15-20 minutes)**: Focus on muscular strength and endurance, as well as core strength with exercises like the "Aqua Crunch" to balance muscle groups in the torso. Use buoyant equipment like handheld aqua bells for alignment and resistance enhancement. Use light hand weights (2-5 pounds) for a revitalizing and uplifting benefit.

4. **Flexibility (5-10 minutes)**: With warmed up tissue, perform static stretches to maintain your joint flexibility, a critical but often neglected component of fitness. To prevent cooling down too rapidly, encourage continuous movement in parts of the body not being stretched—for example, swinging the arms in opposition while performing a calf stretch.

Start where you are. This sample *Splash*Dance format is designed to be inclusive and adaptable; people of all levels of fitness can safely enjoy and benefit from the invigorating world of Aqua-Powered fitness. By considering these elements, you can create engaging, effective, and exceptionally fun training sessions that make you want to come back for more.

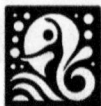

Questions for Reflection and Positive Action

1. **Safety and Standards**: How closely do you align with the American College of Sports Medicine (ACSM) guidelines? Identify your goals and areas for improvement. Plan steps to implement positive and enduring changes.

2. **Customizing Pool Layout**: Considering the layout and characteristics of the pool you use (such as depth, shape, and surface). What new moves and choreography can you try to create adapting to the pool design?

3. **Temperature and Equipment Adjustments**: Evaluate how the water temperature and available equipment currently influence the intensity and enjoyment of your training. What steps can you take to keep warmer?

4. **Creative Use of Pool Edges**: If your pool blueprint allows, design a new routine that incorporates the pool's edge for interval, core, or flexibility training.

PART TWO

Aqua Fitness
Leadership

CHAPTER 30

Commanding the Current - *Splash*Dance Positive Leadership Techniques

Individually we are one drop; together we are an ocean.

- Ryunosuke Satoro

In the vibrant world of aqua fitness, true leadership transcends routine instruction—it thrives on passion, expertise, and a profound commitment to community, all a part of positive leadership.

Introduction to Aqua Fitness Leadership

The aquatic exercise industry is thriving, presenting significant opportunities for fitness professionals. As one of the fastest-growing sectors, aqua fitness is supported by an increasing body of research and increasing participation, underscoring its vast health benefits.

Effective leadership is characterized by a deep understanding of the subject matter, coupled with the ability to communicate clearly and persuasively. A good leader is not only informed but also enthusiastic, injecting humor and personal experiences to make discussions more relatable and engaging. They maintain a poised and confident demeanor, making eye contact and speaking with a lively tone to avoid monotony. Leaders excel by being organized yet flexible, ready to adapt to new challenges as they arise. They create an inclusive environment by being understanding and responsive, listening actively and valuing everyone's contributions without judgment. This approach not only inspires trust and respect but also motivates others to emulate these positive behaviors in professional settings.

For instructors and enthusiasts considering a career in this field, diving into aqua fitness not only diversifies your skill set but also enhances your career longevity and purpose, allowing you to deliver substantial health benefits to a diverse clientele. Within *Splash*Dance, embracing aqua fitness leadership equips instructors to create a dynamic and healthy environment for all.

Sara Palumbo, Director of Aquatics at Neptune (NJ) Aquatics Center since 2009, oversees a world-class natatorium, offering programs that cater to everyone—from children's classes to adult water ballet, team swimming, and a variety of aqua fitness classes. Having participated in classes there for about 10 months, including Deep-Water Running and Aqua Intervals, I've experienced first-hand the diversity and effectiveness of these programs, which range from aqua aerobics to core training and circuit training.

I spoke with Sara about the success and popularity of her aquatics center. She emphasized, "Water Fitness is here to stay. It's accessible to non-swimmers and swimmers alike, and you don't even need to get your hair wet to enjoy a great workout." She also noted the appeal of the "drop-in" nature of the program, which adds to its convenience and popularity. Sara highlighted that the passion and energy of the instructors, who make a point to know participants' names and create a welcoming environment, are key to the program's success. The leadership at Neptune Aquatics Center exemplifies the varied and effective ways to lead in the realm of aqua fitness.

Leading with Heart and a Lot of Fun

Diane Valvo brings over 20 years of fitness leadership experience and an MBA to her role at Neptune Aquatics Center, where her popular classes like "Aqua Deep Water Running and Circuit Training" often have a waiting list. Diane's dynamic personality—athletic, engaging, and with a smile—sets her apart. She exudes positive leadership, ensuring participants feel welcomed, which is fundamental for cultivating a supportive community. Her classes blend challenging exercises with enjoyment, all set to a diverse musical playlist.

In a candid discussion, Diane shared her guiding principle: "It's all about the people." Similar to how I approach my practice, this philosophy shapes the aim to make a meaningful impact on our participants' lives, allying with the foundational principles of effective leadership, a key component of *Splash*Dance.

Diane Valvo's journey offers a blueprint for what it means to lead in the realm of aqua fitness. Her approach aligns with the leadership theory presented in *Splash*Dance, where the fusion of knowledge, inclusivity, and a heartfelt connection to the community sets the stage for a possible transformative aqua fitness experience.

Preparation and Competency Successful aqua fitness instructors need to exhibit a broad array of competencies:

- **Physiological Knowledge**: Proficiency in general fitness, cardiovascular health, muscular strength and endurance, and flexibility is crucial. An understanding of how these elements are influenced by aquatic environments enhances your instruction quality.

- **Anatomical and Safety Expertise**: Knowledge of basic anatomy and kinesiology is essential, along with skills in injury prevention and first aid. Instructors must be able to create safe and effective workout sessions that cater to a diverse population, including older adults, prenatal and postnatal women, individuals with obesity, arthritis, back pain, or those recovering from surgery or injury.

- **Instructional Skills**: Effective aquatic instructors excel in a variety of ways including multi-level and intergenerational teaching, as well as leadership training. They understand how to adeptly monitor and adjust the physical environment as well as the activity in order to suit varied fitness levels and ensure all participants receive optimal benefits. Caring about people, as well as being a good observer and listener, helps build understanding and positive communication.

Teaching *Splash*Dance: Core Principles and Techniques

Teaching *Splash*Dance goes beyond routine instruction; it involves a deep understanding of exercise science tailored to water environments:

- **Educational Foundation**: Instructors need to have a solid grasp of aqua exercise science and physics to apply principles appropriately in water settings.

- **Certifications and Safety**: Possessing training foremost, along with up-to-date certifications in CPR and basic life support are fundamental. Instructors should also be skilled in water safety to quickly address any emergencies or issues that arise during classes.

- **Personalization and Inclusivity**: Effective programming requires adjusting exercises to meet the needs of diverse participants. This includes understanding nutritional basics, exercise modifications, and the use of tools like the Borg scale for rate of perceived exertion (RPE), the Talk Test, to tailor workouts for participants' individual capabilities, goals, and enjoyment.

- **Engagement and Community Building**: Successful instructors not only teach but also engage. Knowing participants' names, understanding about their health histories, and fostering a community atmosphere are key elements that enhance the group fitness experience. Ideally, Instructors are active from both from the deck and in the water, demonstrating exercises and participating alongside attendees to motivate and guide them.

- **Communication and Feedback**: Clear, encouraging communication is essential. Instructors can regularly seek feedback to refine their approach, ensuring that classes meet the expectations and needs of participants while maintaining a focus on fun, safety, and effectiveness.

Cues for Cueing and Non-Verbal Communication

Introduction to Effective Cueing Effective cueing is pivotal in ensuring participants not only understand but also correctly perform aqua fitness exercises. Here are some key strategies for optimizing communication between instructors and participants. These are important in leading a successful and enjoyable class experience, in a place where acoustics are often a challenge.

Essentials of Effective Cueing

1. **Clear and Concise Language**: Utilize straightforward, direct language to communicate instructions. Keep cues brief, focusing on essential actions or modifications, and avoid technical jargon that might confuse participants.

2. **Visual Demonstrations**: Enhance verbal cues with visual demonstrations whenever feasible. Performing the movements yourself helps clarify the intended exercise form and technique and is particularly beneficial in the visually challenging aquatic environment.

3. **Breaking Down Movements**: Make complex exercises into simpler, manageable components. Address each segment sequentially, building from the basic movement to the complete form, which aids in better execution and retention.

4. **Analogies and Imagery**: Employ analogies and descriptive imagery to make movements relatable and easier to visualize. For instance, describe a stride movement as "gliding like a skater on ice," making the abstract motions more tangible.

5. **Sensory Cues**: Apply cues that encourage participants to engage with the water's properties, such as feeling the resistance or sensing buoyancy. These cues enhance proprioceptive awareness and deepen the connection with the exercise environment.

6. **Corrective Cues**: Use constructive feedback to guide proper technique and posture. Phrase cues positively, such as saying, "Keep your spine tall," instead of "Don't slouch," to promote a positive and proactive approach to adjustments.

7. **Repetition and Reinforcement**: Regularly repeat critical cues to reinforce proper techniques and ensure consistent application throughout the session, particularly during transitions between exercises.

8. **Individualized Cues**: Tailor cues to meet individual needs, observing participants for cues that address specific challenges or adaptations. This personalized approach fosters inclusivity and effectiveness.

Cueing with Q-Signs

"Q-signs," or visual cues, are essential non-verbal signals that instructors can use to communicate exercise instructions clearly, especially in noisy environments where auditory cues may be insufficient. Establishing a set of clear, consistent Q-signs improves the understanding and execution of exercises. Effective cueing enhances communication, increases participant engagement, and ensures safety and efficiency during workouts.

Examples of Common Q-Signs:

Q-Sign	Description
Start/Stop	Raise one hand to start an activity. Lower both hands to stop an activity.
Change Direction	Point in the intended direction to guide participants' alignment.
Intensity Levels	Use hand gestures to indicate intensity levels: one finger for low, multiple fingers for higher.
Tempo/Rhythm	Tap a rhythm on your body to align participants with the exercise beat.
Modification Options	Show different hand signals to indicate exercise modifications, accommodating various fitness levels.
Sequence Initiation	Point upwards or to the head to cue the beginning of a sequence, aiding anticipation of transitions.

Before leading a class, introduce your Q-signs to ensure clarity and efficient follow-through. Maintain an encouraging tone, provide ongoing feedback, and be responsive to participants' needs.

To ensure a positive and engaging experience, consider:

- **Clarity and Precision:** Use straightforward language and break down movements for easy understanding.

- **Visual Aids and Demonstrations:** Utilize demonstrations to clarify movements, especially useful in the visually challenging water environment.

- **Adaptability:** Customize cues and exercises to meet individual needs, promoting inclusivity and effectiveness.

Effective leadership and cueing not only improve the safety and enjoyment of the class but also empower participants to maximize their aqua fitness benefits.

Introduction to Aqua Fitness: *Splash*Dance Leadership

Professional aqua fitness instructors are pivotal in creating an engaging and safe environment. They are adaptable, knowledgeable, and skilled in delivering workouts that accommodate diverse abilities, ensuring every participant feels included and capable. The growing popularity of aqua fitness underscores the need for well-trained instructors who can harness the unique benefits of water to foster physical and social well-being.

Appreciative Aqua Leadership

- **Positive Feedback and Reinforcement**: Aim to consistently acknowledge the efforts of your participants, offering sincere encouragement and highlighting their achievements. Try to "catch your students doing something right," and be generous with sincere praise.

- **Adaptability**: Provide variations in exercises to cater to all skill levels, allowing participants to adjust the intensity according to their comfort and capability.

- **Community Building**: Foster a supportive community by learning participants' names and encouraging interaction, which enhances the social experience of your classes.

General Class Recommendations

- **Warmup**: Always start with a thorough thermal warmup to prepare the body for exercise. Use static stretching and ensure participants are gradually brought to a comfortable exercise temperature.

- **Aerobic and Muscle Toning Segments**: Manage transitions smoothly to maintain alignment and avoid injuries. Integrate a range of movements that consider the balance of muscle use and incorporate flexibility training.

- **Cool Down**: Conclude with a cooldown phase that includes stretching to aid in recovery and relaxation.

Choreography Notes and Musical Selections in Aqua Fitness

To design an effective *Splash*Dance playlist, start by aligning your music choices: Begin with energetic, upbeat songs to energize and engage participants during the warm-up, then transition to faster, more intense tracks to match the vigor of high-intensity segments. Ensure each transition between songs is smooth to maintain the flow of movement and energy levels. For cooldowns, select slower, soothing tunes that encourage relaxation and stretching. It's also crucial to consider the musical preferences of your participants; a diverse playlist that spans various genres can cater to a wide range of tastes, enhancing the overall class atmosphere. Be open to feedback and willing to adjust your playlist based on the responses and energy levels you observe in class, in order to make yours as enjoyable and engaging as possible.

Effective Choreography: Ensure that movements are safe, follow the music's rhythm, and design to the mood of the class. Aim for choreography design that's challenging but easy to follow.

Music Selection: Choose music that is dynamic and matches the intensity, tone, and purpose of the training. Music can move you and enhance the overall class atmosphere.

Safety First: Prioritizing Participant Well-Being

- **Water Safety Protocols**: Always check pool accessibility, water temperature, and surface conditions. Ensure the presence of a lifeguard and have an emergency plan in place.

- **Contraindications**: Avoid exercises that involve extreme or unnatural spinal movements, rapid transitions, or any form that could stress the joints or lead to injury.

Water Exercise Leadership and Teaching Techniques

- **Preparation and Communication**: Before class, make announcements about hydration, pacing, and the plan for the session. Use clear and effective cueing, supplemented by visual "Q-signs" to guide participants through each exercise.

- **Feedback and Interaction**: Engage with each participant if possible, offering individual feedback, adjusting techniques as needed, and encouraging peer interactions to build a community atmosphere. Introduce people to each other.

- **Continuous Learning and Adaptation**: Stay informed about the latest in aqua fitness research and techniques. Regularly update your skills and adapt your teaching methods to incorporate new knowledge.

Ensuring a Positive and Safe Class Environment

- **Regular Monitoring**: Watch your students. Observe and remind them to listen to their body, and to keep track of their rate of perceived exertion, or the Talk Test to ensure they are working within safe limits, not too easily and not too hard.

- **Appropriate Aqua Attire**: Recommend wearing suitable attire, including aqua shoes, to improve performance and to promote safety.

Instructors are the cornerstone of a successful aqua fitness program, requiring a blend of technical skill, interpersonal ability, and a deep understanding of the unique dynamics of water-based exercise. By adhering to these guidelines, instructors can ensure that their classes are not only effective but also safe, enjoyable, and inclusive.

Trailblazing and Leading in a New Vibrant Field

As aqua fitness surges in popularity, it presents a unique opportunity for instructors to become trailblazers in this vibrant field. By championing comprehensive training, prioritizing safety, and fostering empathetic connections, you can transform not just your own career but also profoundly impact the lives of your participants. This is your chance to deliver positive experiences that enhance the well-being of individuals of all ages and fitness levels. Embrace the role of a leader in aqua fitness—inspire a community, promote lifelong health, and celebrate the joy of movement. Join us in leading a wave of change that champions health, community, and enduring vitality.

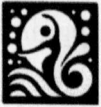

Questions for Reflection and Positive Action

1. **Leadership Philosophy**: How do your personal values and philosophy of leadership align with the positive leadership traits discussed in the chapter?

2. **Community Impact**: In what ways can you, as a leader, foster a sense of community and inclusivity among your participants? Consider how to enhance engagement and connection both during and outside of class sessions.

3. **Professional Development**: What steps can you take to further your education and stay updated with the latest research and techniques in aqua fitness? Reflect on how continuous learning can impact your effectiveness as an instructor and leader.

4. **Safety and Adaptability**: How can you improve safety protocols within your classes to ensure a secure environment for all participants? Additionally, think about how you can better adapt exercises to accommodate your student's diverse needs and abilities.

5. **Feedback and Communication**: What strategies can you implement to enhance communication with your participants, particularly in a challenging aquatic environment? Discuss the importance of observation and positive feedback in refining your teaching methods and class structure.

6. **Personal Reflection**: How has your understanding of effective aqua fitness leadership changed after reading this chapter? Identify any key insights or perspectives that have influenced your approach to teaching and leadership.

7. **Non-Verbal Leadership and Cueing**: How can you effectively utilize non-verbal communication, such as Q-signs, to lead and instruct your aqua fitness classes?

8. **Vision for Leadership**: Looking forward, what is your vision for your role as a leader in the aqua fitness industry? Reflect on how you can use the insights from this chapter to shape a more vibrant, engaging, and health-promoting community.

PART THREE

Aqua Alchemy:
Transformation Toward
Virtue, Flourishing Health,
and Happiness

CHAPTER 31

The *Splash*Dance Leap - Flowing Towards Flourishing

"When you do things from your soul, you feel a river moving in you, a joy." – Rumi

In the pursuit of a good life, the philosopher, Aristotle, spoke of cultivating virtue as essential to human flourishing. This ancient wisdom, emphasizing moral integrity, echoes through time, influencing not only philosophical discourse but also the modern science of positive psychology. *Splash*Dance stands at the crossroads of art and science, serving as a viable social fitness prescription aimed at addressing the challenges of our digital and more sedentary age.

Addressing Modern Challenges with *Splash*Dance

*Splash*Dance effectively, and optimistically, speaks to modern health and well-being challenges like physical inactivity and digital disconnection, while also supporting the "Age Wave," the demographic shift toward an aging population like never before. By encouraging active participation in joyful and socially engaging aquatic exercise, *Splash*Dance aligns perfectly with the principles of aging well and the "autonomy, mastery, and connectedness" associated with positive self-determination, supporting:

- **Physical Health**: Encourages consistent physical activity, and positive movement, enhancing health, well-being, and vitality. Movement matters across the life span and is beneficial to a positively aging society. Positive movement matters and can lead to positive transformation, and vibrant well-being for life.

- **Community Building**: Cultivates a sense of belonging, strengthening social bonds, and combating loneliness and depression.

- **Mental Well-being**: Improves mental health through rhythmic group activities that reduce stress and boost mood with endorphins, alongside brain-building cognitive benefits including mental clarity and executive function.

- **Finding Flow in a World of Digital Disconnection**: Promotes real-world interactions in a safe, fluid environment, providing a healthy counterbalance to increased time on screens. Aqua fitness is a prime place to get into the joy of flow.

- **Inclusivity and Adaptability**: Welcomes individuals of all ages, shapes, sizes, and abilities, fostering a community that respects and appreciates diversity and promotes autonomy, self-efficacy, kindness and caring.

- **Looking at the Big Picture:** "*Splash*Dance is more than just an exercise; it's a movement that champions modern challenges. By training rhythmically in a group, we transcend individual limits and create collective strength, meaning, and goodness. Through mindful attention and unity, we can lead each other towards vibrancy, flourishing health, and positive relationships.

Agency in Action: Building Optimism, Fitness, and Resilience

*Splash*Dance empowers you to recognize and harness   your own capacity to initiate change, both in the water and in your everyday life. This sense of personal efficacy, called agency, is cultivated through each stroke, step, or move, building confidence and resilience. As you experience your ability to influence your physical health, build mental clarity, positive emotions, and social connections, you also develop optimism about your future capabilities. This optimistic outlook, coupled with the imaginative possibilities of achieving personal and communal well-being, transforms *Splash*Dance into a dynamic platform for flourishing, where you are an active agent of your own health and happiness.

*Splash*Dance Promotes Lifelong Learning

*Splash*Dance promotes vital brain health. It also encourages vibrant lifelong learning through several key mechanisms, making it an effective tool for maintaining cognitive vitality as well as physical fitness. Here's an important recap:

1. Cognitive Stimulation Through Choreography Learning:

- Learning and familiarizing yourself with *Splash*Dance moves and steps provides mental stimulation. Each new pattern or sequence challenges the brain, enhancing cognitive function through problem-solving and memory use.

- The process of synchronizing movements with music and adapting to the fluid resistance of water adds an additional layer of complexity, further stimulating neurological pathways.

2. Enhanced Neuroplasticity:

- Regular aerobic activity, such as that provided by *Splash*Dance, is known to increase levels of brain-derived neurotrophic factor (BDNF), a protein that supports the growth of new neurons and the survival of existing brain cells. This contributes to improved neuroplasticity, which is crucial for learning new skills and maintaining cognitive health.

- Engaging in rhythmic, coordinated activities like dance has been shown to enhance the connectivity in brain circuits involved in executive function, motor performance, and multitasking abilities.

3. Reduced Risk of Cognitive Decline and Dementia:

- Studies have shown that physical activities, particularly those involving both aerobic and coordination exercises, can reduce the risk of cognitive decline and dementia. *Splash*Dance, with its dynamic and varied movements, is a potent form of such exercise.

- The social interaction inherent in group dance classes can also help to combat cognitive decline by providing emotional support and reducing stress, which is beneficial for overall brain health.

4. Emotional and Psychological Benefits:

- *Splash*Dance promotes emotional well-being by reducing symptoms of depression and anxiety, which can adversely affect cognitive health. The endorphins released during exercise, combined with the joy of moving and social interaction, contribute to better mood and mental health.

- The aquatic environment itself offers therapeutic qualities, including reduced stress and increased relaxation, which can lead to clearer thinking and better mental performance.

5. Encouragement of a Growth Mindset:

- By continuously offering opportunities to master new skills and improve through practice, *Splash*Dance encourages a growth mindset. This mindset, centered on the belief that abilities can be developed through dedication and hard work, is crucial for lifelong learning.

6. Promotion of Mindfulness and Concentration:

- The focus required to perform aquatic dance moves correctly promotes mindfulness and concentration. These mental skills are beneficial for brain health as they enhance overall cognitive awareness and can stave off mental aging.

By incorporating these elements, *Splash*Dance not only serves as a form of physical exercise but also as a comprehensive cognitive development tool that promotes lifelong learning and supports sustained brain health.

VIA Character Strengths and *Splash*Dance

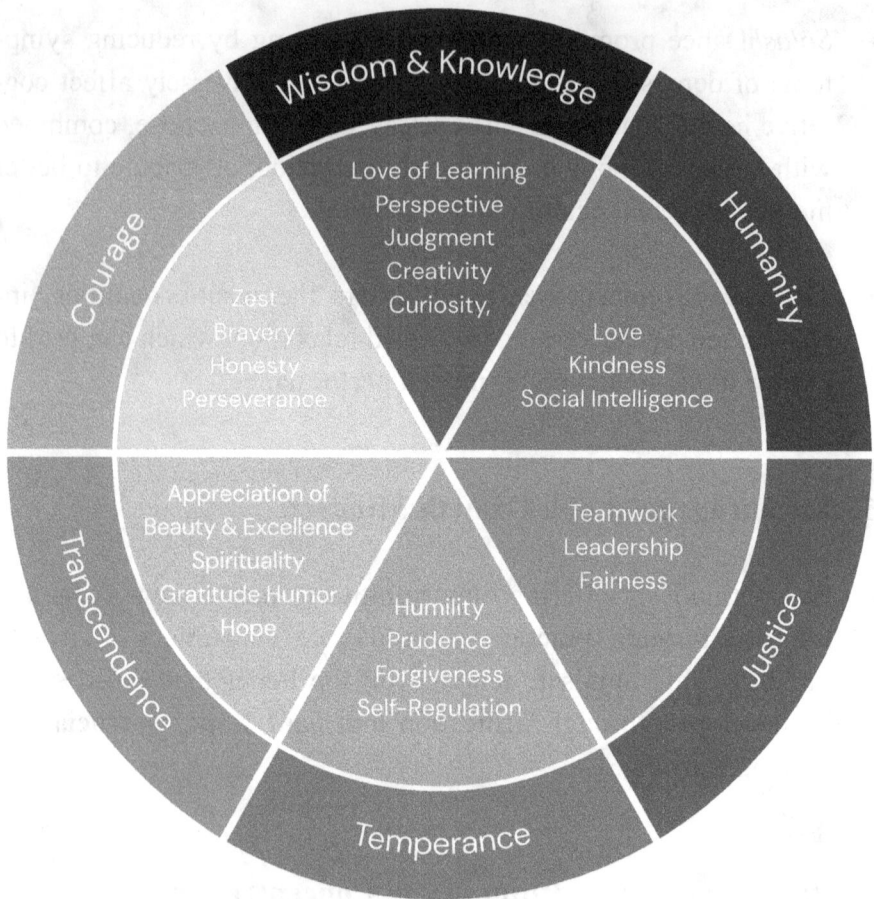

Wisdom & Knowledge

Love of Learning
Perspective
Judgment
Creativity
Curiosity,

Courage

Zest
Bravery
Honesty
Perseverance

Humanity

Love
Kindness
Social Intelligence

Transcendence

Appreciation of
Beauty & Excellence
Spirituality
Gratitude Humor
Hope

Humility
Prudence
Forgiveness
Self-Regulation

Teamwork
Leadership
Fairness

Justice

Temperance

Via Institute on Character (Peterson and Seligman, 2004)

The VIA (Values in Action) Classification of Character Strengths was developed by psychologists Drs. Christopher Peterson and Martin Seligman. The VIA classification is a systematic attempt to identify and categorize positive psychological traits in human beings, often referred to as character strengths. This elegant framework is a cornerstone of positive psychology. The project involved a team of researchers who reviewed a wide range of literature across different cultures, times, and traditions to create a common language of 24 measurable character strengths grouped into these six virtues:

- **Virtue of Wisdom**
- **Virtue of Courage**
- **Virtue of Humanity**
- **Virtue of Justice** (often referred to as Fairness)
- **Virtue of Temperance**
- **Virtue of Transcendence**

These virtues are pathways that can lead us to human flourishing and are integral to developing a full and rich life. The character strengths are important to know and mindfully apply in your life.

*Splash*Dance aligns with the 24 VIA strengths but it seems especially around the Transcendent Strengths—Hope, Humor, Spirituality, Gratitude, and Appreciation of Beauty and Excellence:

- **Hope**: Engaging in *Splash*Dance inspires optimism and motivation for better health and joy, projecting a positive future outlook.

- **Humor**: Light-hearted moments in *Splash*Dance sessions add a layer of enjoyment, making exercise fun and less burdensome.

- **Spirituality**: The soothing presence of water during *Splash*Dance promotes a connection to a deeper, meditative state, enhancing feelings of peace and inner harmony.

- **Gratitude**: Regular participation cultivates a sense of thankfulness for one's physical capabilities and the supportive community environment.

- **Appreciation of Beauty and Excellence**: The elegant and skillful movements performed in *Splash*Dance allow participants to experience and appreciate aesthetic and technical mastery and a magical fluid environment.

By weaving these strengths into the fabric of *Splash*Dance, participants not only improve physically but also enhance their mental and emotional well-being, contributing to holistic well-being.

Call to Action: Embrace the Rhythm of Flourishing

*Splash*Dance is more than an exercise program; it's a vibrant pathway to flourishing that marries ancient wisdom with modern science. Let us move forward together, embracing the rhythms that bind us to build a healthier, happier, more connected, peaceful life and world. Join the dance of life with *Splash*Dance, and let it rejuvenate and inspire you. Embrace the aqua alchemy and transformative power of *Splash*Dance and discover the value and joy it brings. What a feeling!

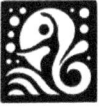

Questions for Reflection and Positive Action

1. **Integration of Virtue and Exercise**: How does *Splash*Dance serve as a platform for cultivating virtue in line with Aristotle's philosophy? Consider and share the specific virtues that you see in yourself.

2. **Digital Disconnection**: In what practical ways does *Splash*Dance help combat the challenges of digital disconnection and sedentary lifestyles? Reflect on your personal experiences.

3. **Aging and Activity**: How does *Splash*Dance address the challenges and opportunities of the "Age Wave"? Consider the program's impact on aging populations in terms of physical health, mental well-being, and social connectivity.

4. **Cognitive Benefits**: Discuss the cognitive and neurological benefits of engaging in *Splash*Dance. How does the combination of physical movement, music, and social interaction contribute to brain health?

5. **Character Strengths and Personal Development**: What VIA Character Strengths resonate with you? Reflect on how these strengths have influenced your personal growth and well-being.

6. **Mindfulness Through Movement**: How does the practice of *Splash*Dance promote mindfulness and

concentration? Share specific instances where you felt these benefits during your sessions.

7. **Emotional Well-being**: *Splash*Dance is said to boost mood and mental health. Discuss how the program has affected and inspired your emotional well-being?

8. **Far-Reaching Positive Aspects**: Looking ahead, what are the far-reaching positive aspects of *Splash*Dance as it continues to evolve? Reflect on its potential impacts on society, health, and education, and how it can continue to influence positive change and policy.

Glossary

Aerobic Endurance: The ability of the heart, lungs, and blood vessels to deliver oxygen to body tissues during sustained rhythmic movement over time.

Agency (Seligman's Perspective): Agency refers to the belief in one's ability to effect change and improve the world. It encompasses efficacy—the confidence in one's capabilities; optimism—the expectation that these capabilities will lead to future success; and prospection—the ability to envision a variety of future possibilities, all fundamental to fostering personal and collective progress.

Agility: The ability to move quickly and easily. Water resistance in *Splash*Dance enhances agility by challenging the body to move against water's viscosity, thus enhancing coordination and speed, including moving in zig zags and grapevines.

Aquatic Barbell: Equipment used in aqua fitness provides added resistance for strength training exercises, increasing the intensity of workouts and range of motion by challenging muscles to work harder against water pressure with more surface area.

Aquatic Therapy Adjustments: Adapting movement and using tools like a flotation belt, noodles, and gloves can support therapeutic needs and rehabilitative goals.

Arm Movements: Specific arm patterns or upper body choreography can enhance the intensity and complexity of aquatic exercises. Varying arm movements can increase or decrease resistance, surface area, and impact, and greatly benefit your training.

Amplitude: Describing large or expansive movements, in *Splash*-Dance, a greater amplitude means that the movements are more pronounced and far-reaching. This can involve the height of jumps, the breadth of arm sweeps, and the distance locomoting.

Bounding Moves: Refers to dynamic movements where both feet leave the ground or pool bottom, during certain jumps or runs. These moves help to increase cardiovascular endurance, muscle strength and bone health.

Buoyancy: A force exerted by a fluid that opposes an object's weight. Buoyancy can provide comfort while reducing strain on the body. This allows you to challenge yourself with exercises that might otherwise be difficult or impossible to do on land.

Cardiovascular Conditioning: Exercises that increase the endurance of the cardiovascular system, allowing the heart and lungs to pump blood and oxygen more efficiently to the muscles during prolonged physical activity. Also called **Aerobics.**

Changing Direction: In water, changing the direction of movement requires additional energy and engages different muscle groups, adding variety and challenge to the exercise routine, thereby enhancing agility, balance, coordination, and the fun factor.

Cognitive Gains: Improvements in brain function and mental capabilities result from regular participation in aerobic activities like *Splash*Dance. Increased blood flow to the brain occurs by nature of the movement, also because it requires coordination and concentration. The music and rhythms contribute to strengthening brain function.

Communitas: A concept of community spirit and social togetherness, fostering a deep sense of connectivity and belonging among participants. This occurs when a group of people are moving in rhythm as one. We become bigger than we are as an individual. Communitas positively supports individual and community well-being over time.

Cooldown: In the final phase of *Splash*Dance, activities are slower and focused on gradually reducing your heart rate, relaxing muscles, centering, and stretching to prevent stiffness and aid in recovery. As you cool down add some stretch intervals: calf stretches, hamstring stretches, quadricep stretches. Hold each stretch 15-20 seconds. Give yourself a big hug, to celebrate your accomplishments and get a nice back stretch.

Cross-Training (CT): A training plan that involves performing and enjoying different types of exercises, or ways to move. CT can promote balanced muscle development, keep up your interest, and improve overall performance by preventing overuse injuries.

Deep-Water Running: Replicating running movements in a deep-water setting, the body is fully suspended, thereby eliminating impact, and allowing for awesome cardiovascular and muscular fitness improvement without joint stress. Recommended to wear a floatation device or use a noodle in order to keep your form and focus.

Drag: Resistance created by moving a body (part) through water. Larger surface areas increase drag, enhancing muscle strengthening, especially during higher speeds.

Eddy: Swirling currents that form around the body or limbs during movement, creating additional resistance and increasing the training intensity. Eddy Resistance adds complexity to the training, requiring more muscle-engagement to maintain stability.

Efficient Muscular Workout: Achieved through the continuous resistance provided by water during deep-water exercises, which engages both upper and lower body muscles, promoting balanced muscle development and endurance.

Enhanced Muscular Balance: In water, exercises benefit from the fluid's multidirectional resistance, which ensures that opposing muscle groups are equally engaged, promoting symmetrical muscle strength, and reducing the likelihood of imbalances.

Flotation Devices: Equipment like belts and noodles that assist in maintaining proper posture, form, and alignment in deep water, allowing for effective full-body benefits.

Fluid Dynamics: The study of fluids in motion. In aqua fitness, understanding fluid dynamics helps you optimize your movements to be more energy-efficient and effective, and utilizing the water's properties to enhance your exercise benefits.

Force Application: The amount of force applied during movements. Greater force increases the intensity and effectiveness of the exercise training.

Frontal Surface Area: The area of the body that faces the direction of movement. Increasing this area increases resistance, making movements more challenging.

***FUNctional* Fitness**: Fitness aimed at supporting and enhancing the performance of everyday activities enjoyably. In *Splash*Dance, functional fitness is achieved through movements mirroring daily actions, enhancing strength, flexibility, and endurance.

Gratitude: In the field of positive psychology, gratitude is regarded as a transcendent strength. It involves recognizing and appreciating the positive aspects of one's life. Within the framework of *Splash*Dance, practicing gratitude can significantly enrich the experience. Engaging in gratitude exercises, such as the "Three Good Things" where you reflect daily on three positive events, can deepen your appreciation, and enhance the overall positive impact of their aquatic fitness journey.

Harmonious Passion: Harmonious Passion refers to a strong inclination towards an activity that one loves and values, which remains under one's control and aligns harmoniously with other aspects of life, leading to positive outcomes such as joy and fulfillment without conflict or stress.

Hydrostatic Pressure: The pressure exerted by a fluid due to its weight. In aqua fitness, deeper water increases hydrostatic pressure, which has benefits such as improved circulation, increased respiratory efficiency, and enhanced joint support.

Impact Manipulation: The technique of adjusting a move's impact forces to meet your fitness level and physical conditions; this allows you to tailor your training plan to your individual needs, ensuring effective training while minimizing the risk of an injury.

Interval Training: A higher level method of training where periods of high-intensity exercise are alternated with periods of lower intensity or rest. This technique is effective in both shallow and deep water, boosting cardiovascular health and metabolic rate. Tabata Training is a challenging and effective form of high-intensity interval training (HIIT).

Kinesthetic Awareness: The enhanced perception of your body position and movement within a space; this is important in deep water where the lack of solid ground requires greater focus and body control.

Lever Lengths in Water: Refers to the use of long and short limb (arm and leg) positions to alter the intensity of exercises in water. Longer levers increase resistance and intensity, while shorter levers decrease it. Understanding lever lengths allows you to tailor your training to your desired performance goals.

Locomotion: Locomotion in water fitness, often referred to as "traveling through the pool," encompasses a variety of dynamic movements aimed at propelling oneself through the water. This includes walking, jogging, running, jumping, and skipping—each offering different levels of intensity and engagement. In designing locomotion exercises, consider the pool's depth and layout.

Muscle Toning: The process of exercising muscles to increase their size, strength, and definition. *Splash*Dance uses the water's natural resistance, and techniques like increasing speed, surface area and levers, to condition and tone your body's muscles.

Neuroplasticity: The brain's ability to change and reorganize itself by forming new neural connections. This can be enhanced through complex, coordinated activities such as aerobics, dance, sport, and formations, as performed in *Splash*Dance,

Neutral Resistance: The equal resistance encountered from all directions, omnidirectionally, in deep water, which promotes muscle strengthening and reduces the risk of muscle imbalance.

Newton's Laws of Motion:

First – Law of Inertia: An object at rest stays at rest, and an object in motion stays in motion with the same speed and in the same direction unless acted upon by an unbalanced force. In water, this principle means that starting or stopping movements requires more effort, enhancing the exercise intensity.

Second – Law of Acceleration: The acceleration, or speed, of an object depends on the mass of the object and the amount of force applied. In aqua fitness, applying more force leads to faster movements against the water's resistance, allowing for variable workout intensity.

Third – Law of Action and Reaction: For every action, there is an equal and opposite reaction. This law is particularly relevant in aqua fitness, where every movement creates a counterforce by the water, providing resistance that helps build muscle strength, endurance, strength, and coordination.

Non-Bounding Moves: Promoting endurance and strength without excessive strain, these are lower impact moves where one foot remains in contact with the pool bottom. This is effective, easier on the joints, and beneficial for recovering from an injury or if you suffer with chronic joint issues.

Non-Impact Environment: Training suspended in deep-water (with a floatation device), fully challenges and supports the body, preventing any harsh impact, thus protecting your joints, and facilitating recovery. A non-impact environment can provide creative higher-intensity training without the associated risks of land-based exercises.

Omnidirectional Resistance: Resistance encountered from all directions in a water environment. This resistance is variable, depending on the speed, your levers, and force of movements, and provides a unique challenge that enhances strength and endurance across multiple muscle groups.

PERMA Theory of Well-Being and Flourishing: An acronym for Positivity, Engagement, Relationships, Meaning, and Achievement; five essential elements of well-being proposed by psychologist Dr. Martin Seligman. *Splash*Dance incorporates these elements to promote holistic health, happiness, and flourishing.

Positive Psychology: The scientific study of what makes life most worth living, focusing on human flourishing, character strengths, and flourishing well-being. It aims to discover and promote factors that allow individuals and communities to thrive.

Power Striding: A dynamic form of walking or jogging in water characterized by long strides that flex and extend the knees and hips, maximizing the use of leg muscles while hands swing at the sides under the water for added resistance and balance. This effective exercise increases cardiovascular fitness and strengthens the lower body.

Proprioception: Mindfulness and a sensory ability to detect the position and movement of your body in space. In aqua fitness, proprioception is challenged and enhanced due to the fluid environment, while improving your balance and coordination.

Psychological Flow: A mental state in which a person performing an activity is fully immersed in a feeling of energized focus, full involvement, and enjoyment in the process of the activity. *Splash*Dance aims to facilitate this state through engaging, rhythmic, and literal-focused "immersion" in enjoyable water exercises to music.

Psychological Well-being: An important concept that includes holistic positive aspects of mental health, such as positive emotions, satisfaction with life, purpose, and fulfillment. *Splash*Dance contributes to this by incorporating positive psychology elements including flow, PERMA, self-determination, gratitude, and social well-being.

Reduced Impact, Increased Buoyancy: Refers to the natural properties of water that reduce the physical impact of exercises on joints and bones, making it ideal for recovery of injuries and chronic joint conditions. Increased buoyancy aids in performing exercises by supporting the body and reducing weight load on the lower extremities.

Resistance: In the context of aqua fitness, resistance is the force that water exerts against a moving object, which helps tone and strengthen muscles.

Resistance Gloves: An effective aquatic tool that increases the surface area of the hands, adding resistance and intensifying upper body workouts and core strength.

Resistance Training: A form of exercise that improves muscular strength and endurance. In *Splash*Dance, the water itself provides resistance, and additional equipment like aqua barbells can be used to increase this effect.

Rhythmic Endurance Exercises: These are activities in *Splash*Dance designed to sustain continuous movement patterns that challenge and improve cardiovascular and muscular endurance over time.

Self-Determination Theory: Self-Determination Theory (SDT) focuses on intrinsic motivation, suggesting that people are most motivated when they feel autonomous, competent, and connected to others. In positive psychology, this theory supports the idea that meeting these core psychological needs can lead to personal growth and greater well-being.

Social Fitness: This refers to the benefits gained from interacting with others in a group setting, which can improve emotional health and foster a sense of community.

Speed: A variable that can be adjusted to increase the intensity of movements in water. Faster movements generate more resistance, enhancing the training challenge.

Stretching / Flexibility: The ability of muscles and joints to move through their full range of motion. SplashDance increases beneficial flexibility by utilizing water resistance and buoyancy, allowing for deeper static and dynamic stretches, along with improved joint mobility to reduce strain.

Surface Area Manipulation: Refers to the technique of altering the size of the body part exposed to water resistance to modify exercise intensity. For example, extending arms during arm circles increases surface area and resistance, enhancing muscular engagement and workout intensity.

Thermal Regulation: The ability of water to help maintain and regulate your body temperature during exercise, preventing overheating and enabling longer, more comfortable workouts.

Thermal Warm-Up: The initial phase of the *Splash*Dance routine, which prepares the body for the more vigorous activity coming by gently increasing heart rate and circulation through easy movements that also warm up the muscles.

Toes-Heels Movement: A technique in water walking where ankles are flexed, and movement alternates between toes and heels to prevent overuse and muscle cramps.

Vertical Aqua Fitness (VAF): An inclusive, effective, and fun-filled *Splash*Dance training method that involves performing exercises in deep or shallow water. This approach utilizes the resistance of water (aqua physics) to enhance fitness while reducing the impact on the joints VAF is excellent for people of a wide range of abilities and ages.

Water Depth: A factor that affects the intensity and impact of exercises. Deeper water increases buoyancy and reduces impact, while shallower water increases resistance and impact, affecting the challenge of movements, and your ability to control them.

Webs: The term "webs" can refer to the natural spread of the fingers that mimics the function of webbed aqua fitness gloves. When you spread your fingers wide during exercises, it increases the surface area of your hands, which adds resistance as you move through the water. This technique helps in strengthening the muscles of your arms and upper body by maximizing the water's resistance.

Thermal Regulation. The ability of water to help maintain and regulate your body temperature during exercise, preventing overheating and enabling longer, more comfortable workouts.

Thermal Warm-Up. The initial phase of the sport/dance routine which prepares the body for the more vigorous activity by gently increasing heart rate and circulation through slow, controlled movements.

[text illegible]

[text illegible]

[text illegible]

[text illegible]

Water. The buffer keeps you cool and provides traction through resistance, gliding water, gradually increasing resistance, which adds resistance to routine. Through the water, the exercise helps in strengthening the muscles of the arm and upper body by maximizing the water's resistance.

References and Resources

Auchauer, H. (2023, July 12). The Full-Body Pool Workout That Doesn't Involve Swimming. The New York Times.

Becker, B. E., & Cole, A. J. (2010). *Comprehensive aquatic therapy.* Butterworth-Heinemann Cooney, G. M., Dwan, K., Greig, C. A., Lawlor, D. A., Rimer, J., Waugh, F. R., ... & Mead, G. E. (2013). Exercise for depression. *Cochrane database of systematic reviews*, (9).

Borg, G. A. (1982). Psychophysical bases of perceived exertion. *Medicine and Science in Sports and Exercise, 14*(5), 377-381.

Buettner, D. (2012). *The Blue Zones: 9 lessons for living longer from the people who've lived the longest.* Washington, D.C.: National Geographic.

Csikszentmihalyi, M. (2020). *Finding flow: The psychology of engagement with everyday life.* Basic Books.

Deci, E. L., & Ryan, R. M. (2021). *Self-Determination Theory: Basic Psychological Needs in Motivation, Development, and Wellness.* New York, NY: Guilford Press.

Dunlap, E., Alhalimi, T., McLaurin, N., & Tanaka, H. (2024). Aquatic Cognitive-Motor Exercise Training on Cognition and Neurotrophic Factors in Older Adults. *Archives of Physical Medicine and Rehabilitation, 105*(4), e180.

Dychtwald, K., & Flower, J. (1989). *Age Wave: How The Most Important Trend Of Our Time Will Change Your Future.* Bantam Books.

Ehrenreich, B. (2006). *Dancing in the Streets: A History of Collective Joy.* New York, NY: Metropolitan Books.

Emmons, R. A. (2021). *The Little Book of Gratitude: Create a Life of Happiness and Wellbeing by Giving Thanks.* London: Gaia.

Fredrickson, B. L. (2009). *Positivity: Groundbreaking research reveals how to embrace the hidden strength of positive emotions, overcome negativity, and thrive.* New York: Crown Publishers.

Fredrickson, B. L., & Joiner, T. (2018). Reflections on positive emotions and upward spirals. *Perspectives on Psychological Science, 13*(2), 194-199. DOI:10.1177/1745691617692106

Hecht, B. J. (1984). *Wet and wonderful water exercises.* Camelback Records & Pub.

Hefferon, K. (2013). *Positive psychology and the body: The somatopsychic side to flourishing.* Open University Press.

Katz, J. (1999). *Aquafit: Water Workouts for Total Fitness.* New York, NY: McGraw-Hill.

Katz, J., Ford, M., & West, J. (1995). The therapeutic effects of water. *Journal of Physical Therapy Science, 7*(1), 1-3.

Kucia, K., Koteja, A., Rydzik, Ł., Javdaneh, N., Shams, A., & Ambroży, T. (2024). The Impact of a 12-Week Aqua Fitness Program on the Physical Fitness of Women over 60 Years of Age. *Sports, 12*(4), 105.

Lianov, L. S., Adamson, K., Kelly, J. H., Matthews, S., Palma, M., & Rea, B. L. (2022). Lifestyle Medicine Core Competencies: 2022 Update. *American Journal of Lifestyle Medicine.* 2022;0(0).

Monroe, M. (2012, August 20). The Happiness Factor, Part One. *IDEA Health and Fitness Association.* Updated October 21, 2013.

Monroe, M. (2012, August 20). The Happiness Factor, Part Two: Learn how to overcome the brain's negativity bias and help your clients move toward joy. *IDEA Health and Fitness Association.*

Monroe, M. (2004). Benefits of water exercise for post-rehab populations. *Journal of Aquatic Physical Therapy, 12*(2), 22-34.

Monroe, M. (2002). *Water Exercise for Therapy and Fitness.* San Diego, CA: Therapy Skill Builders.

Murthy, V. H. (2020). *Together: The healing power of human connection in a   sometimes-lonely world.* Harper Wave.

Nichols, W. J. (2014). *Blue mind: The surprising science that shows how being near, in, on, or under water can make you happier, healthier, more connected, and better at what you do.* Little, Brown Spark.

Niemiec, R. M. (2018). *Character strengths interventions: A field guide for practitioners.* Hogrefe Publishing.

Niemiec, R. M. (2014). *Mindfulness and character strengths: A practical guide to flourishing.* Hogrefe Publishing.

O'Brien, E., & Seydel, A. (2022). *The power of play: optimize your joy potential.* Live Life Happy Publishing.

O'Brien, E. (2019). The rhythm is gonna get you: Music, movement, and positive emotion. *WholeBeing Institute Newsletter.*

O'Brien, E. (2016). Move2Love and vibrancy: Community dance/fitness. *Women & Therapy,* 39(1-2), 171-185. doi:10.1080/02703149.2015.1108392

O'Brien, E. (2014). Positive fitness, movement, and mindful breathing. In M. W. Snyder (Ed.), *Positive health: Flourishing lives, well-being in doctors.* Balboa Press.

O'Brien, E. (2013). *Applying the PERMA Model. IDEA Fitness Journal*

Peterson, C., & Seligman, M. E. P. (2004). *Character strengths and virtues: A handbook and classification.* Oxford University Press.

Putnam, R. D. (2000). *Bowling alone: The collapse and revival of American community.* Simon & Schuster.

Seligman, M. E. P. (2011). *Flourish: A visionary new understanding of happiness and well-being.* Free Press.

Sova, R. (2000). *Aqua Dynamics: The Art and Science of Water Exercise.* Milwaukee, WI: Atrium Publishing.

Ratey, J. J. (2008). *Spark: The revolutionary new science of exercise and the brain.* Little, Brown and Company.

Vallerand, R. J. (2008). On the psychology of passion: In search of what makes people's lives most worth living. *Canadian Psychology/Psychologie Canadienne,* 49(1), 1-13.

Vallerand, R. J. (2015). *On the psychology of passion: In search of what makes people's lives most worth living.* Canadian Psychology/ Psychologie Canadienne, 49(1), 1-13.

Waller, B., Lambeck, J., & Daly, D. (2009). Therapeutic aquatic exercise in the treatment of low back pain: A systematic review. *Clinical Rehabilitation, 23*(1), 3-14.

Westfall, K. (2000). The impact of water fitness on cardiovascular health. *American Journal of Sports Medicine, 28*(5), 672-678.

Acknowledgements, with Sincere Gratitude

Thanks to the lifeguard who saved me when I was 10 at Linden Pool. Thanks to Sean O'Brien, Lianna Marie Tarantin, my Mom, Dad, and Nunni, to whom the book is dedicated. With love for my beloved late "Hall of Fame" and "Teacher of the Year(s), brother, Mike Perrotta. Thanks Debbie Perrotta. Bravo John Brimhall, our son-in-law, who surfed the wave and skated into our hearts. You and your family, Lianna included, are amazing.

Cheers, Andrea Seydel, my book doula, *Live Life Happy* publisher, talented friend, co-author of The Power of Play: Optimize Your Joy Potential.

For Louisa Jewel, MAPP, for being a sister, (dearest friend) & Master Minder, with Coach Extraordinaire and cherished friend, Caroline Adams Miller, MAPP, & world-reknowned, Dr. Margarita Tarragona. What great joy, light, and inspiration each of you are to me.

For our Theano Writer's Workshop, esteemed fellow MAPP members, Jaime Jenkins & (Dr) Lisa Sansom, led by Kathryn Britton. Your talent leaves me in awe as does your kind support and encouragement.

Sending thanks to my PhD advisor, Temple University (TU) Kinesiology, Human Movement Psychology Professor Emeritus, Dr. Michael Sachs, my awesome TU undergraduate students, & fellow TU graduates doing great work.

I am deeply grateful to Professor, Dr. Marty Seligman and the world class faculty at the University of Pennsylvania Masters of Applied Positive Psychology Program (MAPP) program, especially Dr. James Pawelski. Cheers for MAPP Class of 2008. Sending appreciation for my MAPP family, including Karen Deppa, Sharon Danzger, Sandy Blaine,

Sherri Fisher, Ilene Schaefer, Dr. Denise Quinlan, Brian Selander, Cristian Vera, Katie Snyder, Cathy Parsons, Ming Fu, Martha Knudson, Louis Alloro, Kellie Cummings, Vanessa King, Sonya Looney, Paula Toledo, Jennifer Cory, Lara Kallander, Carolyn Biondi, Dr. Gloria Park, Dr. Judy Salzberg, Dr. Lucy Hone, Jenny Brennan Viall, Jodi Wellman, Mariah De Bose, Tamara Myles, Shannon and Jordana's Speakers' Studio, MAPP Master Minders, and the MAPP Alumni, "Body Full of Joy" Team. Thanks to Dr. Scott Glassman, the first Philadelphia College of Osteopathic Medicine MAPP class, and Dr. Eric Langenau.

I extend heartfelt thanks to Dr. Helena Marujo of the University of Lisbon, an international leader, including for IPPA, for her inspiring mission and dedication to peace. Thank for your leadership, Ruth Sova, founder Aquatics Exercise Association, and Dr. Mary Monroe. Thanks to Dr. Liana Lianov, MD.

I am deeply grateful for John Aria, my trusted accountant and long-time friend. Thanks for your guidance, unwavering support and inspiration.

Hug to Carol Dunphy, and Aedan Dunphy, thanks for the bagpipes.

To Treye Blackburn, and his staff at Fairway Mews (FM), Spring Lake Heights, NJ. What a joy to be a part of your team at FM pool for the last 20+ summers, (when we were babies, especially you). Thanks, Barbaran O'Connor, Barbara Blasi, Kay and Ed Christenson, Terry, Peg, Kathleen, Dr. Erin Hartnett, Dr. Susan Reinhart, Noreen Lake, Betty, Ciel, Faye and all our fabulous FM pool *Splash*Dance students. Thank you to each and every one of my land and water dance fitness students. I hold you forever in my heart. Thanks, Karen Lenhart Cook, and athletes, champions, and for National Aerobics Championship Judge's including Carol Boyer and Robbie Raugh. Thank you for your leadership, Kathie and Peter Davis and founding IDEA Health and Fitness Association

Sending my appreciation to Ms. S, to Patty DiPano, and Stephen Mandeville, The Comfort Zone, Ocean Grove, NJ

Thanks Director, Neptune Aquatics Center family, Sara Palumbo, her great staff, along with awesome classmates including Trish, Sharlene, Marianne, Susan Twidle, Kathy Fry, Cheryl Dyer, Mary Kay Seifert, Janet, Trish (from FM), Anne, Diane Valvo, and Liz Arno (for her excellent aerobics, Pilates and yoga class).

Thank you Talia Schatzman, 21 Digby, for your expert administration support and design. Thanks to you my friend, Diane Queen, Trax, and to Nicole and Laurie for all the fun. Thank you Luis Alberto Peña Valdés.

Sean and I are so blessed to have the most wonderful neighbors in historic Ocean Grove, NJ. I'm grateful for Lola, our "island girl" Sato pup from Puerto Rico, who has introduced us to many new friends, and who loves playing with us on the beach.

Thanks to our friends, and readers, including Michelle Barrett, Eli Lilly and Company International Book Club, who enjoyed *The Power of Play*.

Thanks to the fantastic podcasters and interviewers we've met and for every invitation to share with you. What a thrill.

For darling my mother-in-law, thanks for having Sean. Mom Mary Ann, I adore you, your lovely daughters, Alison, Julie, Becky and family.

Thanks to anyone I've forgotten, but who has led me to a path of kindness, wisdom, and understanding.

To my friends, a big hug, with love, Elaine

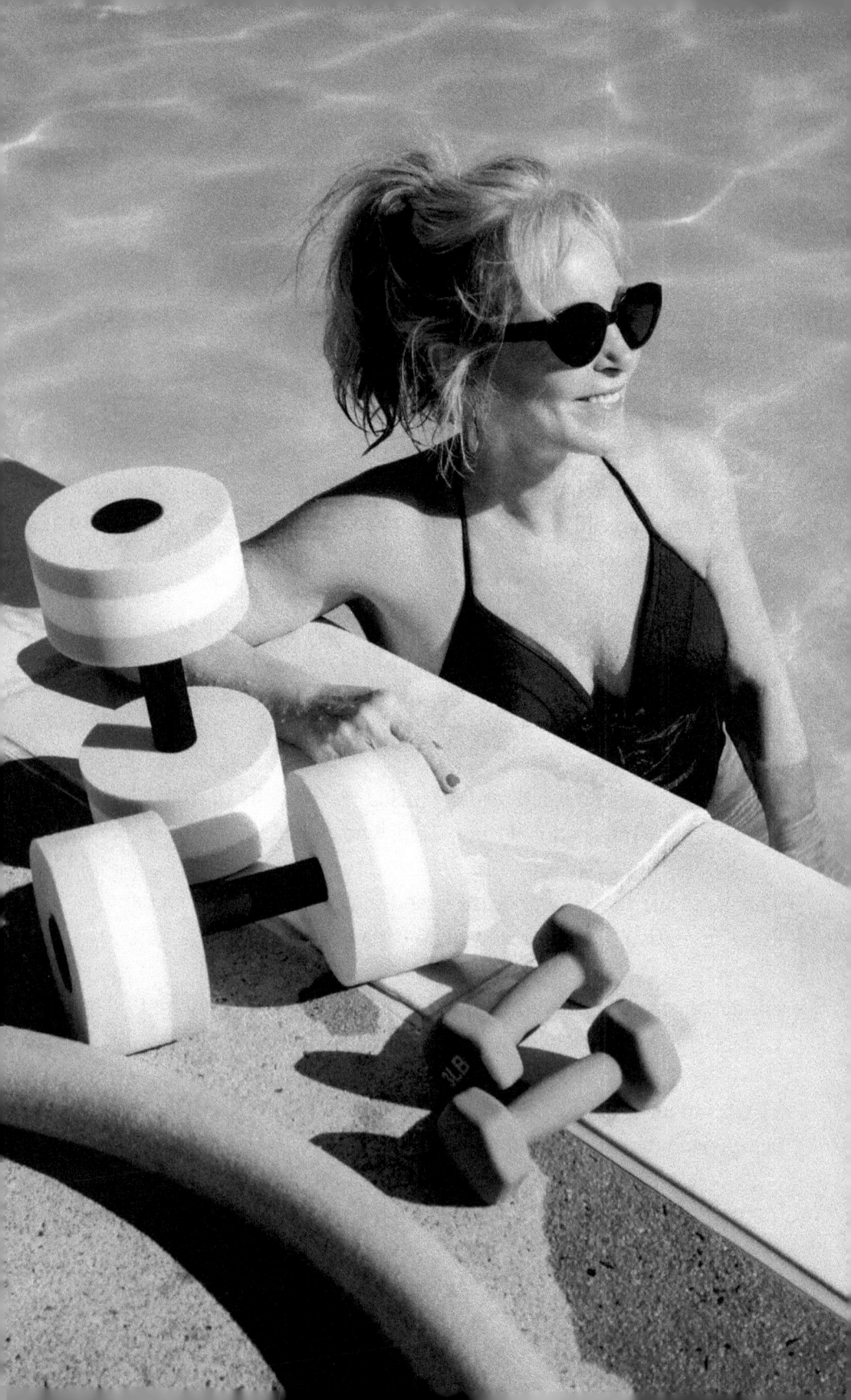

ABOUT THE AUTHOR

Dr. Elaine O'Brien is a passionate champion for optimal health and happiness, seamlessly blending Positive Psychology, Whole Fitness, Dance/Exercise, the Power of Play, and the science of Aqua Dynamics. Globally recognized as a pioneering thought leader, Dr. O'Brien promotes flourishing health and well-being, including through the transformative power of positive movement.

Elaine is among the first 100 graduates of the University of Pennsylvania Master of Applied Positive Psychology (MAPP) program, under Dr. Martin Seligman. She also earned a PhD in Kinesiology, specializing in the Human Movement Psychology, under Dr. Michael Sachs, Temple University, where she also taught Kinesiology: Personal Fitness.

Known for her dynamic presence and engaging leadership style, Dr. O'Brien energizes global audiences with her knowledge, experiences, workshops, and her "Dr. Elaine's Epic Energy Breaks"—melding fitness and fun, with strategic joyful movement and play as essential for individual, corporate, and community thriving. Her aim is to revitalize and connect people to flourishing health.

Dr. O'Brien views water as the ideal medium for holistic health and fitness, welcoming participants of all ages, shapes, sizes, and abilities to experience both gentle and invigorating workouts in the uniquely supportive, healing and empowering environment of water.

As co-author of "The Power of Play: Optimize Your Joy Potential," Dr. O'Brien enriches lives and reshapes our understanding of the interplay between physical and mental health in pursuit of happiness.

Her holistic approach transcends traditional fitness, fostering inspiring leadership and personal growth.

Join Dr. Elaine O'Brien in SplashDance: What a Feeling!, where she infuses her expertise and boundless enthusiasm into a narrative that promises to uplift, inspire, and mobilize you towards a life filled with more health, happiness, and joy.

www.Dr.ElaineOB@gmail.com
www.elaineobrienphd.com
https://www.facebook.com/Elaine.OBrien.Fitstyle
https://www.instagram.com/elaineobrienphd/
https://www.linkedin.com/in/elaine-o-brien-phd/

PRAISE FOR DR. ELAINE O'BRIEN

"Elaine O'Brien has been a pioneer in integrating the worlds of physical movement and positive psychology. She is wise teacher who brings out the best in each person, helping us reconnect with our vitality and with joy in life. What makes Elaine most special for me, is her kindness and huge heart, which are evident from the first time you meet her."

– Dr. Margarita Tarragona, PhD., President, Mexico Positive Psychology Association

"Dr. Elaine O'Brien is one of the most informed, cutting-edge academics in the world on the intersection of the science of happiness and the science of movement. She is one of the first people in the world to get a Master's degree in Applied Positive Psychology (MAPP), and a PhD in exercise science, which sets her apart from others, as does her decades of pioneering work in the power of movement in wellbeing, especially in groups, as well as its legacy effect on families and communities."

– Caroline Adams Miller, MAPP Speaker, Author, Educator, Coach

"Dr. Elaine O'Brien is an international leader in the field of positive exercise and movement and how that contributes to psychological well-being. Dr Elaine's groundbreaking research discovers why physical exercise is a powerful tool for combating depression, anxiety, and loneliness and how it strengthens communities. She is a pioneer in understanding the mind-body connection and offers science-backed strategies that support health, longevity, and well-being. She is definitely my go-to person for everything exercise."

– Louisa Jewell, MAPP, President, Canadian Positive Psychology Association

"Then, and now, your energy, positivity, knowledge, and passion all impressed and inspired me. You are truly a phenomenal scholar and friend."

– Dr. Erica Tibbets, Temple University Co-Researcher, and Smith College

Even more compelling than the movement is the environment Elaine O'Brien creates in her classes. Her positive energy seems to grow out of a mix of her genuine concern for her students, and her serious professional curiosity about the effects of exercise on the whole person throughout her (or his) lifetime...I appreciate the community that Elaine has created and like other artists, I find her original and stimulating to know."

– Dr. Pat Hutchinson, PhD, Fulbright Scholar, Artist, Educator

"Elaine radiates joy and lifts everyone up around her. You cannot buy nor manufacture her potent combination of brains and heart. I have partnered with Elaine on several initiatives. In addition to being an internationally recognized pioneer in the field of exercise medicine and wellbeing, she shares her tremendous knowledge with grace and generosity."

– Jenny Brennan, MAPP, Founder, Ardent Wellbeing, LLC

"Elaine is an amazing university teacher who always makes the day better and happy, no matter what. I learned so much about myself in her Kinesiology classes. She is one of the best teachers ever."

– Anne, Temple University Allied Health/Pre-Med Student

"Elaine O'Brien is a mover and a shaker literally and figuratively. When she enters a room, everything looks brighter and more possible. Her energy breaks remind us that we can approach life's challenges together with our entire bodies moving in synchrony, not just with the heads perched on our shoulders."

- Kathryn Britton, MAPP, Principal, Theano Coaching, LLC

"Elaine O'Brien is incredibly resourceful in the intersection of physical and psychological wellness. She combines scholarship and reliance on evidence-based results with a wealth of diverse experiences and accomplishments. Elaine applies her intelligence, heart, and boundless energy to every project, and she is among the most generous, nurturing people you will ever meet. Let Elaine develop or improve your programs with her unique and energetic approaches."

– Karen Deppa, MAPP, Principal, PilotLight Resilience Resources, LLC

"I am grateful you are our mentor and teacher, Elaine...And every single week, I see your enthusiasm, and I'm reminded how loving and reassuring you make this class...I will never forget how supportive you always are of what each of us have to say. I will never forget the sense of community and friendship you've build among us. Thank you for generously caring about each one of us, and for listening to us.'

- David Kwok, UPenn Positive Psychology Center

"We salute Elaine for her leadership, dedication, and sincerity. Working with Elaine and her team was a meaningful and enjoyable experience and one of the highlights of my professional career with the American Lung Association. "

– James P. Haney, Community Relations Director, Central New Jersey Lung Association, Inc.

"I've known Elaine for years. She is the brightest of lights, has the biggest of hearts, and makes the world-and my life, better! Elaine served as a Recitation Leader for my Positive Psychology class, where she carried out empirical research interventions every week. Elaine earned rave reviews from every student. Her own research is designed to promote optimal health and performance. Elaine has many strengths and a commitment to excellence."

– Dr. Angela Duckworth, PhD., CEO, Character Lab, MacArthur "Genius Award" Fellow, Professor, UPenn

"Elaine is one of the best presenters I've ever seen."

-Melanie Webb, Editor, All Things Healing

ABOUT THE PUBLISHER

Dear Reader,

As you hold this remarkable book in your hands, we want to express our heartfelt gratitude for becoming a part of the Live Life Happy Community of readers. Your curiosity and thirst for knowledge fuel our passion for publishing meaningful non-fiction works.

At Live Life Happy Publishing, our mission is rooted in bringing forth literature that not only entertains but uplifts, supports, and nourishes the soul. We firmly believe that books have the power to transform lives, to ignite passions, and to spread joy far and wide.

Behind every word, every chapter, lies the dedication of our authors who pour their hearts and souls into their craft. Their ultimate aim? To touch your life in profound ways, to inspire, and to leave an indelible mark on your journey.

Your role in this journey is invaluable; by sharing your thoughts through reviews, spreading the word to others, or reaching out to the authors themselves, you become an integral part of sparking transformation in countless lives, igniting a ripple effect of joy and enlightenment.

And if, perchance, you or someone you know has dreams of writing, of sharing a message, or of unleashing a powerful story unto the world, know that Live Life Happy Publishing stands ready to guide you. Our doors are open, our ears attuned, and our hearts eager to hear your message.

So, dear reader, let us, continue to spread the power of literature, one page at a time. Reach out, share, and most importantly, never underestimate the power of your message to touch lives.

With warmest regards,

LiveLifeHappyPublishing.com

P.S. Remember, books change lives. Whose life will you touch with yours?

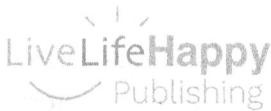

LiveLifeHappy
Publishing

www.ingramcontent.com/pod-product-compliance
Lightning Source LLC
Chambersburg PA
CBHW070756270326
41927CB00010B/2168